AF564558

# Haemoprotozoan Infections in Dairy Animals

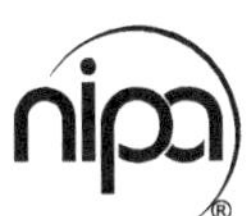

NIPA® GENX ELECTRONIC RESOURCES & SOLUTIONS P. LTD.
New Delhi-110 034

## About the Author

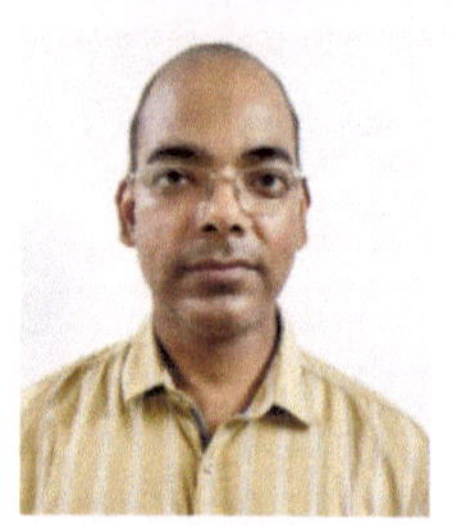

**Dr. Amit Kumar Jaiswal** hails from the Bareilly district of Uttar Pradesh, where he completed his early education. He earned his Bachelor of Veterinary Science and Animal Husbandry (B.V.Sc. & A.H.) degree in 2006 from Chandra Shekhar Azad University of Agriculture & Technology, Kanpur, Uttar Pradesh. Dr. Jaiswal secured the prestigious ICAR-Junior Research Fellowship (JRF) for his Master's program and subsequently completed his M.V.Sc. in Veterinary Parasitology from G.B. Pant University of Agriculture & Technology, Pantnagar, Uttarakhand in 2009. He further advanced his academic credentials by obtaining an in-service Ph.D. in Veterinary Parasitology in 2018. Dr. Jaiswal's professional journey commenced as a Veterinary Officer with the U.P. Government, a role he served from September 2008 to April 2010. He then transitioned to academia, joining the Department of Veterinary Parasitology at the College of Veterinary Science, DUVASU, Mathura, as an Assistant Professor on April 28, 2010, and was subsequently elevated to the position of Associate Professor on April 28, 2023. He is a distinguished lifetime member of several eminent organizations, including the Indian Association for the Advancement of Veterinary Parasitology (IAAVP), The Indian Science Congress Association, Kolkata, and the Indian Society of Veterinary Medicine (ISVM). Dr. Jaiswal has actively engaged in a multitude of trainings, conferences, workshops, and symposia. He also had the honor of being a visiting scholar at the University of Illinois at Urbana-Champaign, Illinois, USA. In recognition of his innovative contributions, Dr. Jaiswal was awarded a patent by the Patent Office, Government of India, as the principal inventor for his creation, "An essential oil-based formulation for control of *Rhipicephalus microplus* tick." His prolific academic output includes six laboratory manuals, numerous popular articles, book chapters, a book, and over 60 research articles published in esteemed national and international journals.

# Haemoprotozoan Infections in Dairy Animals

**Amit Kumar Jaiswal**
Associate Professor
Department of Veterinary Parasitology
College of Veterinary Science and Animal Husbandry
U.P. Pandit Deen Dayal Upadhyaya Pashu Chikitsa Vigyan Vishwavidyalaya Evam
Go-Anusandhan Sansthan (DUVASU), Mathura (U.P.) 281 001

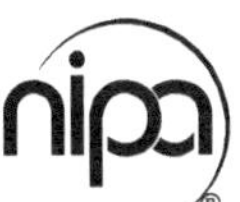

**NIPA® GENX ELECTRONIC RESOURCES & SOLUTIONS P. LTD.**
New Delhi-110 034

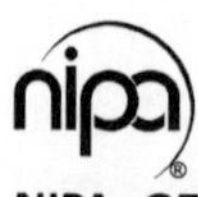

**NIPA® GENX ELECTRONIC RESOURCES & SOLUTIONS P. LTD.**
101,103, Vikas Surya Plaza, CU Block
L.S.C. Market, Pitam Pura, New Delhi-110 034
Ph : +91-11-43860225, Mob.: +91 9717133558, 9540816132
E-mail: newindiapublishingagency@gmail.com
Website: www.nipaersources.com



Print ISBN: 978-93-58873-08-5
ebook ISBN: 978-93-58873-29-0



Composed and Designed by NIPA®.

# Acknowledgements

I first bow my head in reverence to the Almighty God and remain forever grateful for His guidance, immense blessings, and strength in completing this assignment.

It is with great pleasure and deep gratitude that I acknowledge Prof. (Dr.) A. K. Srivastava, Honourable Vice Chancellor, U.P. Pandit Deen Dayal Upadhyaya Pashu Chikitsa Vigyan Vishwavidyalaya Evam Go-Anusandhan Sansthan (DUVASU), Mathura (U.P.) 281 001, and Prof. (Dr.) Vikas Pathak, Dean, College of Veterinary Science & Animal Husbandry, U.P. Pandit Deen Dayal Upadhyaya Pashu Chikitsa Vigyan Vishwavidyalaya Evam Go-Anusandhan Sansthan (DUVASU), Mathura (U.P.) 281 001, for their exemplary leadership, unwavering encouragement, and steadfast support in writing this book.

I extend my heartfelt thanks to the fellow faculty members who contributed to this book, including Dr. Jitendra Tiwari, Dr. Supriya Sachan, Dr. Vivek Agrawal, Dr. Saroj Kumar, Dr. Atul Prakash, Dr. Raju Kushwaha, Dr. Deep Narayan Singh, and others. Their contributions have significantly enhanced the value of this work.

I am also deeply appreciative of the faculty members and associated staff of the Department of Veterinary Parasitology, College of Veterinary Science & Animal Husbandry, DUVASU, Mathura, for their assistance and moral support throughout this endeavour.

Finally, I would like to thank Dr. Kale Chandrakant Dinkar, M.V.Sc scholar from the Department of Veterinary Parasitology and Ishan Garg, 4th Professional B.V.Sc. & A.H. at DUVASU, Mathura, for their contributions to the book chapter and meticulous proof-reading of the book.

**Amit Kumar Jaiswal**

# Preface

The cattle industry faces a substantial risk from haemoprotozoan parasites, which can lead to decreased productivity and increased mortality in dairy animals. Key haemoprotozoa affecting dairy cattle include *Babesia, Theileria*, and *Trypanosoma.* Although the precise financial losses caused by haemoprotozoan infections in dairy animals have not been fully quantified, it is reported that the annual losses attributed to *Theileria parva* alone exceed USD 300 million. Furthermore, parasites such as *Theileria* and *Babesia* are transmitted by tick vectors. In India, the annual financial losses due to tick-borne diseases and tick infestations are estimated at USD 191.15 million. Consequently, it can be inferred that the global annual losses from haemoprotozoan infections likely surpass those associated with tick-borne diseases and the losses from *T. parva* alone.

The primary objective of the book "Haemoprotozoan Infections in Dairy Animals" is to provide a comprehensive discussion of blood parasites affecting dairy cattle. This book addresses important blood parasites, including *Babesia, Theileria*, and *Trypanosoma.* Additionally, it covers significant Rickettsial parasites that may complicate accurate diagnosis by mimicking haemoprotozoa infections. The book also explores crucial topics such as the diagnosis of haemoprotozoa infections, resistance to anti-protozoal drugs, role of nutrition in parasite control, and effective dairy farm management strategies to control these infections.

The author hopes that this book will serve as a valuable resource for veterinary undergraduates and postgraduate students, educators, and veterinary professionals.

**Author**

# Contents

# 1

# General Introduction to Protozoa

***Amit Kumar Jaiswal***

*Department of Veterinary Parasitology, U. P. Pandit Deen Dayal Upadhyaya pashu Chikitsa Vigyan Vishwavidyalaya Evam Go Anusandhan Sansthan (DUVASU), Mathura, Uttar Pradesh*

Protozoa are considered as unicellular eukaryotic organisms and evolved after bacteria and thousands years early to multi-cellular organisms as well as animals. This unicellular eukaryotic organism contains all the organelles or structures like multi-cellular organisms but in single cells. Similar to multi-cellular, the genetic information of protozoa is also stored in chromosomes. The protozoa differ from bacteria in different manners. The differentiating features of bacteria and protozoa are given in Table 1.

**Table 1:** Difference between bacteria and protozoa

| S.No | Characters | Bacteria | Protozoa |
|---|---|---|---|
| 1 | Kingdom | Monera | Protista |
| 2 | Type of organism | Prokaryotic | Eukaryotic |
| 3 | Cell structure | Organelles devoid membrane | Organelles bound with membrane |
| 4 | Cell wall | A peptidoglycan cell wall present | Usually absent |
| 5 | Capsule | Present outside the cell wall or membrane | Absent |
| 6 | Nucleus | No distinct nucleus | Distinct nucleus |
| 7 | Nutrition | Heterotrophic or autotrophic | Heterophytic |
| 8 | Movement | By flagella, cilia or gliding | By flagella, cilia or pseudopodia |
| 9 | Reproduction | Asexual | Asexual or sexual type or both |
| 10 | Size | In micrometers | Micrometer to millimeters |
| 11 | Examples | *Bacillus, Mycobacterium* | *Trypanosoma, Coccidia* |

## 1. General Structures of Protozoa

Protozoa, like other eukaryotic cells, contain a nucleus, endoplasmic reticulum, mitochondria, Golgi apparatus, and lysosomes. Beyond these common organelles, protozoa feature a range of unique structures with specific functions that enable them to operate independently. Protozoan cells can be categorized into two primary components: the cytoplasm and the nucleus.

### Cytoplasm

The cytoplasm of protozoa is a semi-fluid substance enclosed by the cell membrane, housing a variety of organelles such as mitochondria, Golgi apparatus, endoplasmic reticulum, and, in photosynthetic protozoa, chloroplasts. It also includes cytoskeletal elements like microtubules and microfilaments that help maintain cell shape, facilitate movement, and organize internal structures. The cytoplasm is essential for numerous cellular functions, including metabolism, protein synthesis, molecule transport, and support for cellular activities. It is generally divided into two main regions: ectoplasm and endoplasm.

**Ectoplasm:** This is the outer, more gel-like layer of the cytoplasm. It often contains structures involved in movement, such as pseudopodia—temporary extensions used for locomotion and feeding—and sensory structures for environmental interaction.

**Endoplasm:** The inner, more fluid-like region of the cytoplasm contains various organelles necessary for metabolic processes, digestion, and other cellular functions, including mitochondria, Golgi apparatus, endoplasmic reticulum, and food vacuoles.

In addition to these types, other variations of cytoplasm are found in different protozoan groups:

**Hyaline Cytoplasm:** This clear, transparent cytoplasm lacks distinct granules or inclusions. It is often observed in free-living or parasitic protozoa, where it may help with camouflage or evade host immune detection.

**Granular Cytoplasm:** In this type, visible granules or particles are dispersed throughout the cytoplasm. These granules may serve as storage for nutrients, waste products, or other essential substances.

**Synergetic Cytoplasm:** In some colonial protozoa, such as certain flagellates or ciliates, individual cells may share cytoplasmic connections through structures like cytoplasmic bridges or syncytia. This interconnected cytoplasm supports communication, coordination, and resource sharing among the colony's cells.

These cytoplasmic types illustrate the diverse adaptations and functions of protozoa, reflecting their wide range of environments and lifestyles.

## Nucleus

The nucleus in protozoa is a membrane-bound organelle that houses the cell's genetic material in the form of chromosomes. As the control center of cellular activities, the nucleus coordinates gene expression, DNA replication, and cell division. The structure and organization of the nucleus can vary among different protozoan groups and species. Key components of the protozoan nucleus include:

**Nuclear Envelope:** The nucleus is encased by a double membrane known as the nuclear envelope, which separates it from the cytoplasm. The envelope contains nuclear pores that regulate the exchange of molecules, such as RNA and proteins, between the nucleus and cytoplasm.

**Chromatin:** Inside the nucleus, DNA is organized into chromatin, a complex of DNA and histone proteins. Chromatin can be in a condensed form (heterochromatin) or a less condensed form (euchromatin), reflecting different levels of gene activity.

**Nucleolus:** Some protozoa have a distinct nucleolus within the nucleus where ribosomal RNA (rRNA) synthesis occurs. The nucleolus is crucial for assembling ribosomes, which are essential for protein synthesis.

**Nucleoplasm:** The semi-fluid matrix inside the nucleus is called nucleoplasm. It contains various proteins, enzymes, and nucleic acids that are vital for nuclear functions.

**Nuclear Organization:** The organization of the nucleus can vary, with some protozoa featuring multiple nucleoli, indicative of active rRNA synthesis, or a single large nucleolus, depending on the species and its metabolic needs.

Protozoa, being a highly diverse group of unicellular organisms, exhibit considerable variability in nuclear structure and organization. Understanding these characteristics sheds light on their cellular biology, gene expression, and evolutionary relationships.

Protozoan nuclei can generally be classified into two types: vesicular nucleus and compact nucleus. The main differences between these types are summarized in Table 2.

**Table 2:** Difference between vesicular and compact nucleus

| S.No | Features | Vesicular nucleus | Compact nucleus |
|---|---|---|---|
| 1 | Morphology | Appears as dispersed, vesicle-like structures within the nucleus | Appears as condensed, dark-staining structures within the nucleus |
| 2 | Chromatin Structure | Chromatin dispersed or vesicle-like | Chromatin condensed and tightly packed |
| 3 | Function | Primarily involved in gene expression and regulation | Primarily involved in storage and transmission of genetic material |
| 4 | Presence | Found in certain protozoa, particularly ciliates | Found in various eukaryotic organisms, including plants, animals, and fungi |
| 5 | Transcription | Rapid transcription and gene expression occur | Transcription may occur, but typically at a slower rate compared to vesicular nuclei |
| 6 | Replication | Replicates during vegetative growth and undergoes frequent DNA rearrangements. | Replicates during cell division through mitosis or meiosis, maintaining the original genetic material. |
| 7 | Examples | Macronucleus of ciliate protozoa | Nucleus of other protozoa |

## Other Structures of Protozoa

### Locomotory Structures

Protozoa exhibit a variety of locomotory structures, each adapted to their specific environments and ecological niches. The main types of locomotory organs in protozoa include:

1. **Flagella**: These are long, whip-like appendages extending from the cell surface. They move in a whip-like fashion, propelling the protozoan through its environment. Flagella are characteristic of many protozoa, including flagellates like *Euglena* and *Trypanosoma.*

2. **Cilia**: Short, hair-like projections that cover the cell surface in dense rows or patches. Cilia beat in a coordinated rhythm, enabling the protozoan to move or create water currents to bring food particles toward it. Ciliates such as *Paramecium* and *Stentor* are well-known for their ciliary locomotion.

3. **Pseudopodia**: These are temporary, foot-like extensions of the cell membrane used for movement. Protozoa that utilize pseudopodia, known as amoeboid protozoa, move by extending and retracting these projections. Examples include *Amoeba proteus* and *Entamoeba histolytica.*

4. **Undulating Membrane**: Some protozoa have specialized membranes that undulate or ripple, aiding in movement. For instance, the flagellate *Trichomonas vaginalis* features an undulating membrane that produces wave-like movements to propel the organism.

5. **Gliding Mechanisms**: Certain protozoa glide or crawl along surfaces by secreting substances such as mucus or adhesive materials. This mode of locomotion is seen in various protozoa, including some flagellates and ciliates.

**Kinetoplast**: Found in kinetoplastids such as *Trypanosoma* and *Leishmania*, the kinetoplast is a unique organelle located near the base of the flagellum. It contains a complex network of circular DNA molecules known as kinetoplast DNA (kDNA), which is essential for mitochondrial DNA replication and maintenance. The kinetoplast's distinct DNA arrangement plays a critical role in the cell's energy metabolism and has become a target for drug development against kinetoplastid-caused diseases like African sleeping sickness and Chagas disease.

**Chromatoid Body**: This organelle is present in certain protozoa, notably in some ciliates like *Paramecium*. The chromatoid body is a dense, granular structure within the cytoplasm, often near the nucleus. It consists of ribonucleoprotein complexes that are involved in RNA processing, storage, and regulation. The chromatoid body plays a role in synthesizing, modifying, or sequestering RNA molecules and may be prominent during stages of sexual reproduction, cyst formation, or in response to environmental stressors.

These diverse locomotory and specialized structures highlight the adaptability and complexity of protozoa, reflecting their varied ecological roles and evolutionary adaptations.

## 2. Mode of Nutrition in Protozoa

Protozoa exhibit various nutritional modes, primarily categorized into three main types:

- **Holozoic Nutrition**: In this mode, protozoa ingest solid food particles, which are then broken down internally through digestion. This type of nutrition is observed in many animals and certain protozoa. The ingested food is processed within specialized digestive compartments or vacuoles.

- **Holophytic Nutrition**: This mode is characteristic of organisms that perform photosynthesis to produce their own organic nutrients. Also known as autotrophic nutrition, holophytic nutrition involves the synthesis of organic compounds from inorganic substances, using light energy captured by pigments such as chlorophyll. This type of nutrition is found in photosynthetic protozoa, which can convert light energy into chemical energy through the process of photosynthesis.

- **Saprozoic Nutrition**: Protozoa that exhibit saprozoic nutrition obtain nutrients by absorbing dissolved organic matter from their environment. These organisms, including certain flagellates and amoebas, absorb organic molecules like sugars and amino acids directly through their cell membranes. Unlike holozoic protozoa, saprozoic protozoa do not actively capture or hunt prey but rely on the availability of dissolved nutrients in their surroundings.

In addition to these primary modes, protozoa can also exhibit

- **Parasitic Nutrition**: Parasitic protozoa feed on host tissues, bodily fluids, or blood. Examples include *Plasmodium*, which causes malaria, and *Trypanosoma*, responsible for sleeping sickness. These protozoa derive nutrients by exploiting their hosts, often causing disease in the process.
- **Mixotrophic Nutrition**: Protozoa with mixotrophic nutrition utilize a combination of nutritional strategies. For example, some photosynthetic protozoa can also adopt a heterotrophic mode of nutrition when conditions are not conducive to photosynthesis. This flexibility allows them to adapt to varying environmental conditions by switching between autotrophy and heterotrophy as needed.

### 3. Locomotion in Protozoa

Protozoa employ various locomotory structures and mechanisms that are adapted to their environments, evolutionary backgrounds, and habitat characteristics. The primary types of locomotion in protozoa include:

- **Pseudopodia**: Protozoa such as amoebas move using temporary cytoplasmic extensions known as pseudopodia. These projections are formed by the flow of cytoplasm, allowing the organism to extend and retract these projections for movement. This process enables amoeboid protozoa to crawl along surfaces and engulf food particles.
- **Flagella**: Protozoa like *Euglena* and *Trypanosoma* utilize long, whip-like appendages called flagella. Flagella beat in a coordinated, wave-like fashion to propel the organism through liquid environments, such as water.

- **Cilia**: Protozoa such as *Paramecium* possess numerous short, hair-like projections called cilia that cover their surfaces. These cilia beat in a synchronized, rhythmic pattern, generating currents that facilitate movement through their aquatic habitats.
- **Gliding**: Some protozoa are capable of gliding along surfaces. This form of locomotion often involves the secretion of mucous or adhesive substances that reduce friction and help the organism adhere to and move along the substrate.
- **Muscle-like Contractions**: Certain protozoa have contractile fibers or structures that enable them to contract and extend. For example, in some ciliates, the contraction and relaxation of contractile vacuoles assist in movement as well as osmoregulation.
- **Hydrostatic Pressure**: In some amoeboid protozoa, locomotion is facilitated by changes in hydrostatic pressure within the cell. This internal pressure allows the organism to push against its surroundings and move effectively.

## 4. Respiration in Protozoa

Protozoa exhibit various respiratory strategies tailored to their environmental conditions and metabolic requirements. The primary methods of respiration in protozoa include:

- **Diffusion**: Most protozoa utilize simple diffusion for gas exchange. Oxygen from the surrounding environment diffuses directly through the cell membrane into the cell, while carbon dioxide, a by-product of metabolism, diffuses out of the cell.
- **Body Surface Exchange**: Protozoa often have a high surface area-to-volume ratio, which facilitates efficient gas exchange through their cell membrane. This method is especially common in protozoa with a thin or flattened morphology, such as amoebas and certain flatworms, which maximizes the surface available for gas exchange.
- **Anaerobic Metabolism**: In environments where oxygen is scarce, some protozoa can switch to anaerobic metabolism to produce energy. This process typically involves fermentation, where organic compounds are partially oxidized to generate ATP and produce by-products like ethanol or lactic acid.

## 5. Excretion in Protozoa

Excretion in protozoa involves the removal of metabolic waste products to maintain cellular function and osmotic balance. Despite their simplicity as single-celled organisms, protozoa have developed various mechanisms to manage waste, as they lack specialized excretory organs found in more complex organisms. Common methods of excretion in protozoa include:

- **Diffusion**: Similar to gas exchange, small waste molecules, such as ammonia and carbon dioxide, are expelled from the cell through simple diffusion across the cell membrane. This method is particularly prevalent in aquatic protozoa, where waste products readily diffuse into the surrounding water.
- **Contractile Vacuoles**: Freshwater protozoa use contractile vacuoles to regulate osmotic pressure and remove excess water from the cell. These vacuoles actively accumulate water and dissolved waste products, then expel their contents by contracting and fusing with the cell membrane, effectively removing the waste from the cell.
- **Gut Excretion**: Protozoa with a digestive cavity or cytostome (cell mouth) excrete waste products into their digestive vacuoles or gut. These waste-filled vacuoles eventually fuse with the cell membrane, expelling the waste products from the cell as part of the digestion process.
- **Storage as Crystals or Granules**: Some protozoa store metabolic waste products, such as uric acid or calcium carbonate, as insoluble crystals or granules within specialized organelles. These waste products can be periodically expelled from the cell or retained until the organism's death, depending on the species and environmental conditions.

## 6. Reproduction in Protozoa

Protozoa exhibit diverse reproductive strategies, including asexual, sexual, and a combination of both types of reproduction. Here's an overview of these reproductive modes:

### Asexual Reproduction

- **Binary Fission**: This is the most prevalent method of asexual reproduction among protozoa. In binary fission, a single cell divides into two daughter cells, each inheriting a complete set of genetic material. This method is commonly observed in protozoa such as amoebas and paramecia.

- **Multiple Fission**: In multiple fission, a single protozoan cell divides simultaneously into several daughter cells. This process can lead to the formation of multiple offspring within a protective cyst or covering. For instance, the protozoan *Plasmodium*, which causes malaria, undergoes multiple fission within the host's red blood cells.
- **Spore Formation (Sporogony)**: Certain protozoa produce resistant structures known as spores as part of their reproductive cycle. These spores, such as cysts in the genus *Giardia*, are capable of surviving adverse environmental conditions and facilitate dispersal to new habitats.
- **Schizogony (Merogony)**: Schizogony involves multiple rounds of nuclear division (mitosis) followed by cytoplasmic division, resulting in the production of several daughter cells, known as merozoites. This form of reproduction is typical in parasitic protozoa, especially within the phylum Apicomplexa, such as *Plasmodium* species.
- **Budding**: In budding, a new individual forms as an outgrowth or bud on the parent organism. Over time, this bud enlarges and eventually detaches from the parent to become a separate, fully independent organism.

### Sexual Reproduction

- **Syngamy (Fertilization)**: Syngamy is the fusion of two gametes to form a zygote, marking the start of sexual reproduction. In protozoa, this process involves the merging of two haploid gametes, which can be of different mating types or sexes, resulting in the formation of a diploid zygote.
- **Conjugation**: Conjugation is a form of sexual reproduction observed in certain protozoa, particularly ciliates like *Paramecium*. During conjugation, two mating cells exchange genetic material, leading to genetic recombination and increased genetic diversity among the offspring.

These reproductive strategies highlight the adaptability and evolutionary diversity of protozoa, enabling them to thrive in various environments and conditions.

## 7. Classification of Protozoa

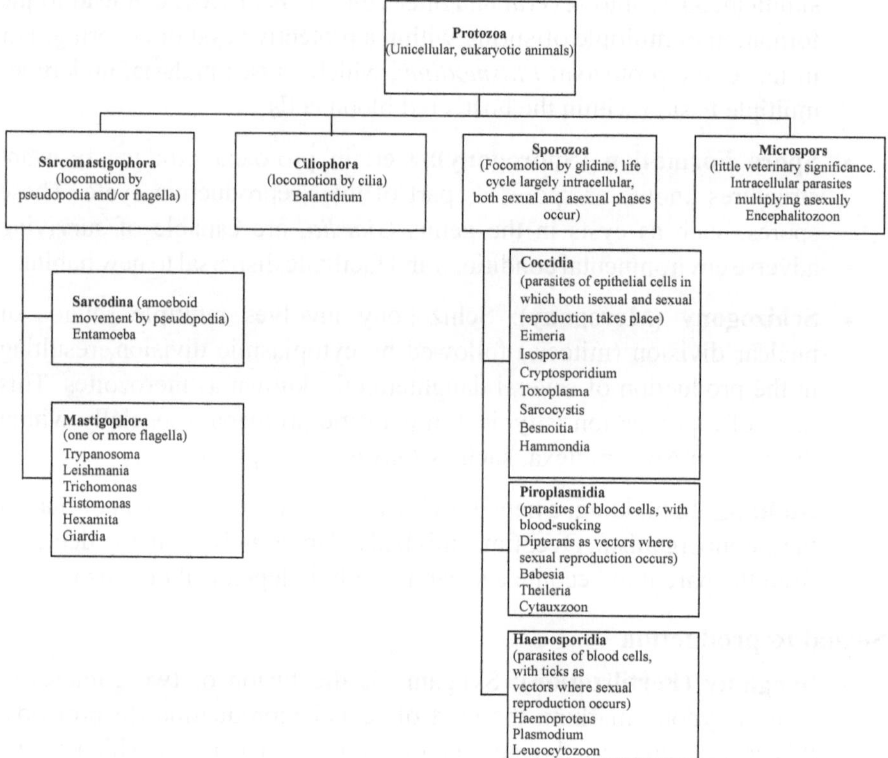


## 8. General Lifecycle of Protozoa

**Direct lifecycle:** A lifecycle that involves only one host for completion. In a direct life cycle, there is no requirement for an intermediate host or vector for the protozoa to complete their lifecycle. This simplicity in transmission often correlates with a more straightforward infection cycle and fewer steps in the transmission process.

Direct lifecycle typically includes the following stages:

### 1. Trophozoite Stage

- The active, motile feeding stage of the protozoa.
- Trophozoites feed, grow, and reproduce by binary fission within the host's tissues or lumen of the organ they inhabit.

### 2. Multiplication and Reproduction

- Trophozoites multiply by dividing into two daughter cells through binary fission.

- This process allows the protozoa to increase their numbers within the host.

**3. Encystation (optional)**

- Some protozoa in direct life cycles may form cysts under adverse conditions, such as to survive outside the host during environmental stresses or to facilitate transmission.

**4. Transmission**

- Transmission occurs directly from one host to another, typically through ingestion of infective stages (e.g., cysts or trophozoites) in contaminated food, water, or from direct contact with infected individuals.
- Ingestion of the protozoa allows them to enter the host's digestive tract and initiate infection.

**5. Development within the Host**

- Once inside the host, cysts may excyst (break open), releasing trophozoites that colonize and multiply in the host tissues or lumen of the organ they infect.
- Trophozoites continue the lifecycle by feeding, growing, and reproducing within the host, perpetuating the infection.

Examples of protozoa with direct life cycles include

- ***Giardia lamblia***: Causes giardiasis in various animals, including humans. It has a direct life cycle involving cysts that are ingested and develop into trophozoites in the small intestine.
- ***Entamoeba histolytica***: Causes amoebic dysentery in humans and other animals. It has a direct life cycle where cysts are ingested and develop into trophozoites in the large intestine.
- ***Tritrichomonas foetus*:** Causes trichomoniasis, primarily a sexually transmitted infection in bovines. It has a direct life cycle where trophozoites are directly transmitted during sexual contact.

**Indirect lifecycle:** An indirect lifecycle in animal protozoa typically involves multiple hosts or stages outside the primary host. This complexity often includes various developmental stages and sometimes requires an arthropod vector for transmission. Indirect lifecycles in protozoa often involve complex interactions between hosts and vectors, allowing for adaptation to different environments and enhancing their transmission capabilities. A general outline of an indirect lifecycle in veterinary protozoa involves:

**1. Definitive Host**

- The primary host where the protozoa undergoes sexual reproduction or reaches sexual maturity.

**2. Vector**

- An additional host required for the completion of part of the lifecycle. This host typically harbors a developmental stage or serves as a vector for transmission to the definitive host.

**3. Lifecycle Stages**

- **Trophozoite Stage**: The active, motile feeding stage of the protozoa that occurs within the definitive host. Trophozoites may cause disease and reproduce asexually.
- **Cyst Stage**: A dormant, resistant stage that allows survival outside the host. Cysts are often involved in transmission between hosts and are typically ingested to initiate infection in the definitive host.
- **Vector**: In cases where a vector is involved, such as mosquitoes or flies, they play a crucial role in transmitting the protozoa between hosts. The protozoa may undergo specific developmental stages or reproduce sexually within the vector.

**4. Transmission**

- Transmission may occur through ingestion of cysts or trophozoites (direct transmission) or through the bite of an infected vector (vector-borne transmission).

**5. Development and Pathogenesis**

- Upon ingestion by the definitive host, cysts may excyst (break open), releasing trophozoites that colonize tissues and cause disease.
- Trophozoites may undergo asexual reproduction within the definitive host, leading to clinical symptoms and disease manifestations.
- In cases where a vector is involved, the protozoa may undergo additional developmental stages within the vector before becoming infective to the definitive host.

Examples of protozoa with indirect lifecycles include

- ***Plasmodium* spp.**: Malaria parasites that infect various animals via mosquito vectors. They require both a vertebrate (definitive) host and a mosquito (vector) host for complete lifecycle.

- ***Trypanosoma* spp.**: Causes diseases like African Trypanosomiasis (Sleeping sickness) and Nagana in animals. They require tsetse flies as vectors for transmission between hosts.
- ***Toxoplasma gondii***: Causes Toxoplasmosis in various animals, including cats and livestock. It has an indirect lifecycle involving cats as definitive hosts and various intermediate hosts (e.g., rodents, birds).

## 6. Mode of Transmission of Protozoa

### 1. Ingestion of cysts or trophozoites

- Many protozoa have environmentally resistant cyst stages that are shed in feces or other bodily fluids of infected animals.
- Transmission occurs when these cysts or trophozoites are ingested by a susceptible host through contaminated food, water, soil, or direct contact with infected individuals.
- Example: *Giardia* spp., which causes giardiasis in animals including dogs and cats, is transmitted through ingestion of cysts shed in feces.

### 2. Vector-Borne Transmission

- Some protozoa require an intermediate vector (such as mosquitoes, flies, or ticks) to complete their lifecycle and transmit between hosts.
- The protozoa develop within the vector, which becomes infected by feeding on an infected host, and then transmit the protozoa to a new host during subsequent feedings.
- Example: *Plasmodium* spp., which causes malaria in birds and mammals, requires mosquitoes as vectors for transmission.
- The vector borne transmission is of different type; Cyclical or biological, Non-cyclical or mechanical, trans-ovarian and trans-stadial or stage to stage transmission.

### 3. Direct Contact

- Direct contact between infected and susceptible animals can transmit protozoa that are shed in bodily fluids or trans-stadial through close contact.
- This mode is common in sexually transmitted protozoal infections or infections spread through direct contact with infected tissues or secretions.

- Example: *Tritrichomonas foetus*, which causes bovine trichomoniasis, is transmitted through direct contact during mating or through contaminated instruments.

**4. Vertical Transmission**

- Transmission of protozoa from a pregnant female to her offspring, either transplacentally (across the placenta) or during parturition (birth).
- This mode ensures the protozoa's continuation within the population without requiring external transmission factors.
- Example: *Toxoplasma gondii*, which causes toxoplasmosis, can be transmitted vertically from a pregnant female to her offspring.

**5. Fomite Transmission**

- Transmission through contaminated objects or fomites (e.g., bedding, equipment) that carry infectious cysts or trophozoites.
- Animals can become infected by coming into contact with contaminated surfaces or objects.
- Example: Protozoa like *Cryptosporidium* spp. can be transmitted through contaminated water or surfaces in animal facilities.

**6. Venereal Transmission**

- Some protozoa, particularly those affecting reproduction or in genital tract transmit during sexual intercourse from male to female or vice versa.
- *Tritrichomonas foetus* in bovines and *Trypanosoma equiperdum* in equines are the examples.

## References

Acharya, R. (2015). Protozoan Diversity in India's Biodiversity Hotspots. Jaipur: Vikas Publishing House.

Adams, R.J. (2015). Introduction to Protozoology. 3rd ed. London: Springer.

Adams, S.L. (2019). Protozoa in Microbial Ecosystems. New York: McGraw-Hill.

Anand, R.K. (2015). Protozoan Biology: Indian Perspectives. New Delhi: Tata McGraw-Hill.

Baker, H.K. & Green, M. (2018). Fundamentals of Protozoa Biology. Oxford: Oxford University Press.

Baker, M.E. (2015). Medical Protozoology: A Clinical Approach. Oxford: Oxford University Press.

Banerjee, A. & Choudhury, R. (2018). Protozoa and Parasites in India. Kolkata: Oxford University Press.

Bhatnagar, R. (2016). Protozoa and Disease Transmission in Indian Context. New Delhi: Jaypee Brothers Medical Publishers.

Bhattacharya, S. (2016). Protozoa and Waterborne Diseases in India. New Delhi: Narosa Publishing.
Carter, A.D. & Evans, M.L. (2021). Applied Protozoology. 3rd ed. San Francisco: Freeman.
Carter, D.J. (2021). Protozoology: A Comprehensive Guide. New York: McGraw-Hill.
Chakraborty, S. (2016). Fundamentals of Protozoology. 2nd ed. Mumbai: Pearson.
Chatterjee, P. (2018). Protozoan Biology for Indian Students. 2nd ed. Kolkata: Academic Publishers.
Das, A. (2017). Protozoology and Public Health in India. Hyderabad: Pearson India.
Davies, L. (2019). Protozoa: Microscopic Creatures of the World. Chicago: University of Chicago Press.
Dawson, F.J. (2018). Protozoan Physiology and Function. 2nd ed. London: Wiley-Blackwell.
Desai, P. & Joshi, A. (2019). Protozoa: Ecology and Diversity in Indian Waters. New Delhi: Academic Press.
Dutta, S. (2019). Protozoa in Indian Soil Ecosystems. Hyderabad: Orient Blackswan.
Edwards, P.A. & Harris, S.G. (2017). Protozoa in Water Treatment Systems. New York: Academic Press.
Evans, W. & Clarke, J. (2014). Cellular Life and Protozoa. Cambridge: Cambridge University Press.
Ford, L.J. (2014). The Protozoan Kingdom. Boston: Pearson.
Ford, T.A. (2016). Protozoology Explained. 2nd ed. Edinburgh: Elsevier.
Ghosh, M. (2021). Protozoology: Research and Development in India. Chennai: Jaypee Brothers Medical Publishers.
Ghosh, P. (2021). Protozoa in Indian Agriculture. Bangalore: Wiley India.
Gopal, K. (2019). Protozoan Parasites in Indian Communities. Bengaluru: Narosa Publishing.
Grant, H.P. (2020). Protozoology in Medicine and Health. 4th ed. Oxford: Oxford University Press.
Green, M.L. (2020). Advanced Protozoology Studies. Boston: Pearson.
Hill, G.A. & Thompson, S. (2017). Protozoan Ecology and Evolution. New York: Wiley.
Hill, J.T. & Morgan, C.S. (2016). Protozoan Pathogens: A Biological Overview. New York: McGraw-Hill.
Iqbal, Z. & Khan, S. (2017). Protozoa and Indian Agriculture. New Delhi: Tata McGraw-Hill.
Irvine, D.K. (2013). Protozoa: A Microscopic World Unveiled. Cambridge: Cambridge University Press.
Irvine, P.R. (2013). Protozoa in Medical Research. London: Academic Press.
Iyer, M.K. (2017). Medical Protozoology in India. 3rd ed. Chennai: Jaypee Brothers Medical Publishers.
Jain, S.K. (2020). Protozoology: A Guide for Students. New Delhi: Tata McGraw-Hill.
Jenkins, R.T. (2019). Environmental Protozoology. 2nd ed. London: Springer.
Jenkins, S. & Morgan, R. (2020). Protozoology in Modern Science. San Francisco: Freeman.
Johnson, R.T. (2015). Protozoa: Unicellular Wonders. New York: Academic Press.
Kapoor, A.R. & Singh, R.K. (2014). Protozoa in Indian Freshwater Ecosystems. Hyderabad: Orient Blackswan.
Karlson, J.P. & Reed, B.A. (2016). Protozoa in Human Disease. 2nd ed. London: Wiley-Blackwell.
Kaur, R. (2016). Protozoa in Indian Water Bodies. New Delhi: Jaypee Brothers.
Kent, S.L. & Moore, A.J. (2021). Protozoa: Cellular Organization and Behavior. San Francisco: Freeman.

Khan, A. (2018). Protozoology: A Comprehensive Indian Textbook. Mumbai: Academic Press.
Kumar, D. (2018). Protozoa and Human Health in India. Mumbai: Academic Publishers.
Lal, P. & Bhatia, V.K. (2016). Protozoa in Environmental Science: Indian Perspectives. Kolkata: Springer India.
Lawrence, P.H. (2014). Essentials of Protozoology. 3rd ed. Boston: Pearson.
Lewis, P.C. (2015). Protozoan Reproduction and Evolution. New York: Academic Press.
Maheshwari, N. & Reddy, P. (2020). Protozoan Parasites in Indian Fisheries. Chennai: Pearson India.
Malhotra, S. (2015). Protozoan Studies in Indian Wildlife. New Delhi: Narosa Publishing.
Martin, J.W. & Brown, A. (2017). Protozoa: Form and Function. Oxford: Oxford University Press.
Mehta, S. (2014). Protozoan Studies in Indian Ecosystems. New Delhi: Tata McGraw-Hill.
Miller, A. (2017). Protozoa and Their Environments. Oxford: Oxford University Press.
Nair, P.R. & Rajan, K.C. (2021). Introduction to Protozoa: An Indian Approach. Chennai: Tata McGraw-Hill.
Nanda, R.K. (2015). Protozoa and Human Diseases in India. Hyderabad: Academic Publishers.
Narayanan, S. & Pillai, G. (2021). Protozoan Parasites in Indian Wildlife. Bengaluru: Orient Blackswan.
Nelson, L.B. (2020). Protozoan Life Cycles and Their Environment. 2nd ed. Cambridge: Cambridge University Press.
Newton, C.L. (2021). The Protozoan World: A Microscopic Perspective. Cambridge: Cambridge University Press.
Oliver, J.P. (2019). Introduction to Protozoan Biology. London: Springer.
Olson, H.P. (2018). The Protozoan Cell: A Study in Complexity. London: Academic Press.
Pandey, A. (2019). Protozoan Parasites in Indian Livestock. Jaipur: Vikas Publishing House.
Patel, J. & Deshmukh, S. (2017). Protozoa in Indian Wetlands. Kolkata: Academic Press.
Peterson, K.F. & White, D.L. (2018). Protozoology for Beginners. San Francisco: Freeman.
Quinn, D.J. (2019). Protozoology: Ecology, Behavior, and Evolution. New York: McGraw-Hill.
Quinton, R.J. (2016). Protozoa in Marine Ecosystems. 2nd ed. New York: McGraw-Hill.
Rao, S.K. (2017). Protozoology for Medical Students in India. 2nd ed. Bengaluru: Wiley India.
Rao, V.K. (2018). Protozoa in Indian Coastal Ecosystems. Chennai: Tata McGraw-Hill.
Rogers, M.K. (2013). The Role of Protozoa in Ecology. Edinburgh: Elsevier.
Rogers, P.F. (2016). Protozoa in the Food Chain. Oxford: Oxford University Press.
Roy, M. & Sen, S. (2020). Advanced Protozoology: Research in India. Kolkata: Academic Press.
Saxena, A. (2020). Medical Protozoology in India's Public Health Sector. New Delhi: Jaypee Brothers.
Sharma, D. (2016). Protozoa and Disease Transmission in India. New Delhi: Jaypee Brothers.
Sharma, P. & Gupta, R. (2019). Protozoan Studies in India's River Systems. Mumbai: Pearson India.
Sharma, R. & Singh, S. (2020). Protozoa in Indian Agricultural Practices. New Delhi: Academic Press.
Singh, A. (2018). Protozoa in Indian Marine Ecosystems. Mumbai: Orient Blackswan.
Singh, D. (2016). Protozoan Parasites of Indian Domestic Animals. Kolkata: Academic Press.
Sinha, P. & Patel, R. (2019). Protozoology: Indian Contributions to Science. Hyderabad: Academic Publishers.
Stevens, H.L. & Turner, P.A. (2020). Protozoa: Diversity and Adaptation. 3rd ed. Boston: Pearson.

Stewart, E.M. (2014). Protozoan Parasites of Humans and Animals. 3rd ed. London: Springer.
Subramanian, G. (2021). Protozoan Pathogens in Indian Agriculture. Chennai: Pearson India.
Taylor, N.G. (2018). Protozoa: The First Eukaryotes. Oxford: Oxford University Press.
Thakur, R. (2018). Protozoa in India's Forest Ecosystems. New Delhi: Narosa Publishing.
Thompson, J.L. & Davis, R.M. (2021). Protozoa in Soil Ecosystems. New York: Wiley-Blackwell.
Tiwari, S. (2014). Protozoa in Indian Rivers and Lakes. New Delhi: Tata McGraw-Hill.
Tripathi, M. (2021). Protozoan Pathogens in Indian Public Health. Hyderabad: Academic Publishers.
Underwood, S.J. & Walsh, R.T. (2021). Protozoan Parasites and Human Health. New York: Academic Press.
Upadhyay, S. & Gopal, R. (2017). Protozoa and Infectious Diseases in India. Bengaluru: Jaypee Brothers Medical Publishers.
Upton, R.J. (2017). Protozoan Biology: Principles and Practice. Boston: Pearson.
Vaughan, M.K. (2015). The Role of Protozoa in Disease Transmission. Cambridge: Cambridge University Press.
Venkatesh, R. (2019). Protozoan Parasites in Indian Freshwater Ecosystems. New Delhi: Orient Blackswan.
Verma, N.K. (2017). Medical Protozoology in Indian Context. 3rd ed. New Delhi: Wiley India.
Verma, P. (2015). Protozoology: An Indian Perspective. Chennai: Tata McGraw-Hill.
Vincent, P.E. (2015). Protozoology in Environmental Science. Cambridge: Cambridge University Press.
Watson, J.K. (2019). The Life Cycle of Protozoa. 2nd ed. London: Academic Press.
Williams, B.L. (2020). Protozoology: The Hidden World. 2nd ed. London: Wiley-Blackwell.
Xavier, L.R. & Young, C. (2016). Protozoa and Infectious Disease. Oxford: Oxford University Press.
Yadav, R. & Mishra, V.K. (2020). Protozoa and the Indian Environment. Kolkata: Academic Press.
Yadav, S. (2018). Protozoan Diseases in Indian Livestock. Mumbai: Vikas Publishing House.
Young, M.J. (2017). Protozoan Studies in Modern Biology. New York: Wiley-Blackwell.
Zane, P.F. & O'Connor, M. (2019). Protozoan Diversity in Freshwater Ecosystems. New York: Academic Press.
Zaveri, H. & Desai, A. (2020). Protozoan Diversity in India's Wetlands. Kolkata: Academic Press.
Zimmerman, T.L. (2014). Protozoology: Key Concepts and Methods. Boston: Pearson.

Stewart, R. M. (2014). *Protozoan Parasites of Humans and Animals*. 3rd ed. London: Springer.
Subramanian, G. (2021). *Protozoan Pathogens in Indian Agriculture*. Chennai: Pearson India.
Taylor, N.C. (2018). *Protozoa: The First Eukaryotes*. Oxford: Oxford University Press.
Thakur, R. (2018). *Protozoa in India – Forest Ecosystems*. New Delhi: Narosa Publishing.
Thompson, J.L. & Davis, K.M. (2020). *Protozoa in Soil Ecosystems*. New York: Wiley-Blackwell.
Tiwari, S. (2019). *Protozoa in Indian Rivers and Lakes*. New Delhi: Tata McGraw-Hill.
Tripathi, M. (2021). *Protozoan Pathogens in Indian Public Health*. Kolkata: Academic Publishers.
Underwood, S.J. & Walsh, R.P. (2021). *Protozoan Parasites and Human Health*. New York: Academic Press.
Upadhyay, S. & Gopal, [illegible] (2017). *Protozoa and Infectious Diseases in India*. Bengaluru: Jaypee Brothers Medical Publishers.
Upton, R.J. (2017). *Protozoan Biology: Principles and Practice*. Boston: Pearson.
Vaughan, M.K. (2015). *The Role of Protozoa in Disease Transmission*. Cambridge: Cambridge University Press.
Venkatesan, R. (2019). *Protozoan Diversity in India's [illegible] Ecosystems*. New Delhi: Orient [illegible]
Verma, [illegible] (2017). *Medical Protozoology* [illegible]
Verma, P. (2018). *Protozoology: Applied* [illegible]
Vincent, P.L. (2015). *Protozoology and Environmental Science*. [illegible] University Press.
Watson, T.K. (2019). *The Life Cycle of Protozoa*. 2nd ed. London: Academic Press.
Williams, S.T. (2020). *Protozoology: The Hidden World*. 2nd ed. London: Wiley-Blackwell.
Xavier, L.R. & Young, C. (2016). *Protozoa and Infectious Diseases*. Oxford: Oxford University Press.
Yadav, R. & Mishra, V. (2020). *Protozoa and the Indian Environment*. Kolkata: Academic Press.
Yadav, S. (2018). *Protozoa and their Role in Indian Livestock*. Mumbai: [illegible] Publishing House.
Young, M.T. (2017). *Protozoan Studies in Modern Biology*. New York: [illegible]
Zhu, L. & O'Connor, [illegible] (2019). *Protozoan Diversity* [illegible] Academic Press.
Zweig, H. & Dean, [illegible] (2020). *Protozoan Diversity* [illegible] Press.
Zimmermann, H. (2011). *Protozoology: Key Concepts and Methods*. Boston: Pearson.

# 2

# Trypanosoma

***Amit Kumar Jaiswal[1], Aditika Singh[1] and Amit Singh[2]***

*[1]Department of Veterinary Parasitology, U. P. Pandit Deen Dayal Upadhyaya Pashu Chikitsa Vigyan Vishwavidyalaya Evam Go Anusandhan Sansthan (DUVASU), Mathura-281 001, Uttar Pradesh*
*[2]Department of Veterinary Parasitology, Acharya Narendra Deva University of Agriculture And Technology, Kumarganj, Ayodhya-224 229, Uttar Pradesh*

Kingdom: Protozoa

Phylum: Euglenozoa

Class: Kinetoplasta

Order: Trypanosomatida

Family: Trypanosomatidae

Genus: *Trypanosoma*

Members of the genus *Trypanosoma* are responsible for trypanosomosis in animals and human beings and are found in the blood vascular system and tissues all over the world. All the species of trypanosomes are transmitted biologically or mechanically through an arthropod vector except *T. equiperdum*, which is transmitted through coitus in equines.

## Morphology

Trypanosomes are leaf-like or sometimes rounded body organisms having a vesicular nucleus. Several sub-pellicular microtubules are found below the outer membrane. A single flagellum arises from the basal body. A variable undulating membrane attaches the flagellum with the outer membrane making the flagellum free or fixed in different species of trypanosomes. A rod-shaped or spherical kinetoplast with DNA is present posterior to the basal body. The members of this family are originally parasites of the intestinal tract of insects. Members of the genus *Trypanosoma* are heterogeneous with amastigote, promastigote, epimastigote and tryptomastigote stages in their life cycle. Generally, trypomastigote stages are found in the vertebrate host. In typical

**tryptomastigote** form, the kinetoplast and basal body are found near the posterior end and the flagellum arises from the basal body and attaches with undulating membrane that extends along the side of the body to the anterior end. In the **epimastigote** form, the kinetoplast and basal body are just posterior to the nucleus and the undulating membrane runs forward from there. The **promastigote** form, the kinetoplast and the basal body are anterior in the body without an undulating membrane. In the **amastigote** form, the body is rounded in shape and a short flagellum emerges from the body.

## Transmission

All trypanosomes except *T. equiperdum* required arthropod vectors for transmission from one animal to another. The transmission of trypanosomes is divided into cyclical and non-cyclical.

***Cyclical transmission:*** The cyclical transmission also called as **biological transmission**. In cyclical transmission, trypanosome before forms an infective stage for next susceptible host, it multiplies, undergo a series of morphological transformations in arthropod vector. The cyclical transmission can be either anterior station development or posterior station development. If trypanosomes multiply in the digestive tract and proboscis and new infection is transmitted through proboscis during feeding is known as anterior station development. The group of trypanosomes those develop through anterior station development comes under Salivaria. Trypanosomes transmitted by *Glossina* sp., show anterior station development. The important examples are *Trypanosoma congolense* (subgenus Nanomonas), *T. vivax* (subgenus Duttonella) and *T. brucei* (subgenus Trypanozoon). In few trypanosomes, multiplication and morphological transformation occur in the gut and the infective stages migrate to the rectum and are passed with the faeces called posterior station development. The group of trypanosome species show posterior station development come under Stercoraria. The important examples are relatively non-pathogenic trypanosomes of animals *T. theileri* and *T. melophagium*. Beside these in humans *T. cruzi* is also transmitted through faeces of reduviid bugs comes under stercoraria.

***Non□cyclical transmission:*** The non-cyclical transmission is also called as mechanical transmission. In non-cyclical transmission trypanosomes are transferred from one host to another by the interrupted feeding of biting flies, Tabanids and *Stomoxys* without any multiplication and morphological transformation in vector. The most important example of non-cyclical transmission is *Trypanosoma evansi*, widely distributed in animals of Africa and Asia.

In Central and South America, *T. evansi* is also transmitted by the bites of vampire bats in which the parasites multiply and survive for a long period. This is more than mere a mechanical transmission, since the bat is also a host, although it is certainly non-cyclical, since there is absence of morphological transformation in multiplying trypanosomes in the blood of bats before they migrate into the saliva. The salivarian trypanosomes, normally transmitted cyclically in *Glossina* fly, but may be transmitted mechanically also. The dogs, cats and wild carnivores may become infected by consuming infected carcasses with trypanosomes in which the parasites enter in circulation by oral abrasion.

**Genus: *Trypanosoma:*** Various species of *Trypanosoma* found in animals and man and are transmitted cyclically or non-cyclically. *Trypanosoma* stage found in mammalian host is tryptomastigote and multiply by longitudinal binary fission.

## Cyclically or Biologically Transmitted Trypanosomes

### Salivarian trypanosomes

Salivarian trypanosomes have an elongated body, 8.0 to 39 μm long and the blunt posterior end. A flagellum arises at the posterior end of the trypanosome from a basal body at the foot of a flagellar pocket. The flagellum runs to the anterior end of the body and is attached along its length to the pellicle to form an undulating membrane. *T. brucei*, *T. congolense* and *T.vivax* are the three most important salivarian cyclically transmitted trypanosomes affecting dairy animals in *Glossina* prevalent areas of the world. The important morphological difference among these trypanosomes is given in Table 2.

**Table 2:** Important morphological differences in important salivarian trypanosomes.

| S.No | Characters | *T. brucei* | *T. congolense* | *T.vivax* |
|---|---|---|---|---|
| 1 | Prevalence | Less common | Most common | Less common |
| 2 | Morphology | pleomorphic | monomorphic | monomorphic |
| 3 | Size | <39μm (long and slender form)<br><8μm (short and stumpy form) | 8.0 to 18μm | 20 to 27μm |
| 4 | Undulating membrane | conspicuous | inconspicuous | inconspicuous |
| 5 | Kinetoplast | small and sub-terminal | medium-sized and marginal | large and terminal |
| 6 | Posterior end | pointed | blunt | broad and rounded |
| 7 | Free flagellum | Well developed in slender form Short or absent in stumpy form | no free flagellum | short free flagellum |

| S.No | Characters | *T. brucei* | *T. congolense* | *T. vivax* |
|---|---|---|---|---|
| 8 | Movement | moves rapidly within small areas of the microscope field | moves sluggishly, often apparently attached to red cells | moves rapidly across the microscope field |

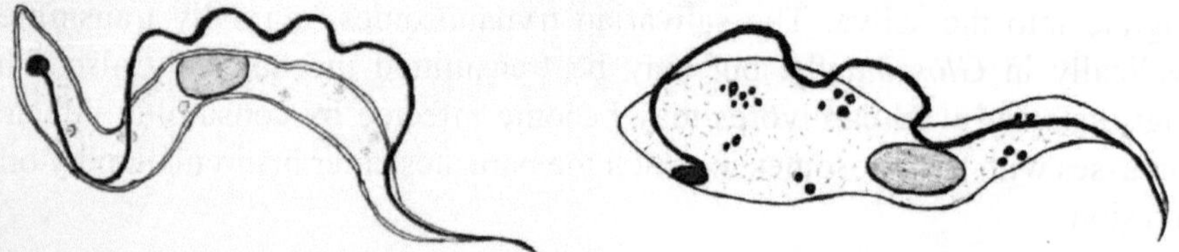

**Fig. 2.1:** *Trypanosoma brucei* **Fig. 2.2:** *Trypanosoma congolense*

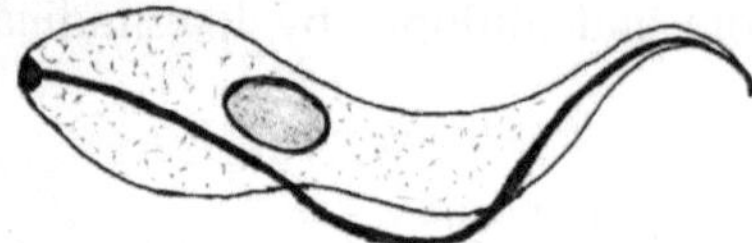

**Fig. 2.3:** *Trypanosoma vivax*

## Life cycle of Salivarian Trypanosomes

Trypanosomes are ingested by tsetse fly during blood feeding on infected host. Trypanosomes lose their glycoprotein surface coat and transform into the epimastigote stage from trypanomastigote stage and start to multiply in the midgut. Thereafter, they reach to proboscis (*T. congolense*) or salivary gland (*T. brucei*) of fly and further transform in trypanomastigote stage with glycoprotein surface coat. In *T. vivax* the complete process of multiplication and morphological transformation takes place in proboscis of fly. These are considered as infective stage of trypanosomes for next susceptible host called as metacyclic trypanosomes. The entire process of development of metacyclic trypanosome takes two to three weeks. The susceptible host becomes infected by inoculation of metacyclic trypanosomes during blood feeding of tsetse fly. At the site of inoculation on host, the trypanosome start multiplying locally and thus a raised cutaneous inflammatory swelling appeared called chancre. After that trypanosomes enter into blood stream and multiply. The parasitaemia is appears in peripheral blood after 1 to 3 weeks and persists for months if untreated.

### Pathogenesis of Salivarian Trypanosomes

The pathogenesis of trypanosomes can be categorize under three heads.

1. ***Lymphoid enlargement and splenomegaly:*** The presence and multiplication of parasites in body of host induce hyper-gamma-globulinaemia especially IgM and plasma cell hyperplasia. After some days because of infection for long duration the lymphoid system become exhausted and there is shrunken of lymphoid organs and spleen.
2. ***Anaemia:*** It is cardinal feature of haemoprotozoa infection including Trypanosomosis. The flagellar movement of trypanosomes causes destruction of RBCs and the destructed RBCs are removed from the circulation by the mononuclear phagocytic system.
3. ***Cell degeneration and inflammatory infiltrates:*** *Trypanosoma* infected animals show cell degeneration in many organs most prominent in skeletal muscles, cardiac muscles and central nervous system. There is separation and degeneration of muscle fibers are reported prominently in cardiac muscles.

### Stercorarian Trypanosomes

#### *Trypanosoma theileri*

**Morphology:** This is a large size trypanosome of about 60–70 μm in length, but may be up to 120 μm. The posterior end is long and pointed. A medium-sized kinetoplast present at posterior end. Undulating membrane is prominent and a free flagellum present. The tryptomastigote and epimastigote forms found in the blood.

**Life cycle:** Multiplication occurs in the vertebrate host by longitudinal binary fission. The trypanosomes develop into small metacyclic tryptomastigotes stages in the hindgut of tabanid flies. Infection occurs in the host by the presence of trypanosomes in the faeces of flies deposited on mucous membranes.

**Pathogenesis:** *T. theileri* is a non pathogenic trypanosome.

### Mechanically Transmitted Trypanosomes

#### *Trypanosoma evansi*

*Trypanosoma evansi* has the widest host range among all trypanosomes. *T. evansi* has a wide geographical distribution that covers all over the world. The disease caused by *T. evansi* is termed as “surra”. It is a complex of diseases induced by a “group” of parasites named *Trypanosoma evansi* (also known as *Trypanosoma brucei evansi*).

## Transmission

*T. evansi* can transmit mechanically through the bite of insects, blood-sucking insects, and also by vampire bats. The transmission can also be reported through vertical, horizontal, iatrogenic, and per-os. Transmission through buffalo leech (*Hirudinaria manillensis*) has also been reported in Asia.

The mechanical transmission of *T. evansi* by biting insects or flies is the most important mode of transmission in dairy animals as well as other livestock and camel also. In early 18$^{th}$ century it was suspected that there may be role of biting flies in transmission of this parasite and called as El debab (means fly) in Algeria and makhi ki bimari (means fly disease) in the Punjab region of India and Pakistan.

Biting flies interrupt by host to have blood meal on an infected host after biting, thus flies off from the host and land on another animal to start its blood meal again. During the first attempts of fly to feed on blood on infective host, the fly mouthparts partially filled with a small amount of blood via capillary action. This residual blood in mouth part of fly partially inoculated into another susceptible animal in the next attempt to bite. Thus the interrupted feeding habbit in flies play important role in *T. evansi* transmission. The estimated blood in proboscis of fly by capillary action in first attempt of bite is 1–12 nl in Tabanids and 0.03 nl in *Stomoxys*. A mathematical model suggested that for a significant transmission of *T. evansi* in a cattle should have a mean burden of 20–30 Tabanids and parasitaemia of above $10^6$ trypanosomes/ml of blood. Literature suggested that the role of *Haematobia* and *Hippobosca* can not be ignored flies for transmission of *T. evansi*. Trypanosomes survive in biting flies for a short time for example *T. vivax* in tabanid fly survives only for 30 minutes and 10 to 15 minutes in *Stomoxys*. So, the infection is possible if the lapse between two interrupted blood is a less than 30 minutes. Thus, in a herd or large number of animals in an area, there may be more chance of successful transmission. *T. evansi* in insect gut or crop get the suitable environment for survival and can survive for 5 to 7 hours. Tabanid and *Stomoxys* are the prime biting flies for transmission of *T. evansi*. However, few reports showed the role of Culicidae and Ceratopogonidae in trypanosome transmission mechanically. Experimentally, *T. evansi* successfully transmitted by *Aedes aegypti*, *Aedes argenteus* and *Anopheles fuliginosus*. Sucking flies like *Musca* sp. can also transmit trypanosomes by contamination of wound. For example, *Musca crassirostris* was reported for transmission of *T. evansi*. In some situation sucking flies may increase the risk of mechanical transmission of *T. evansi* by transfection. Briefly, sucking flies like *Musca* sp. on the body of cattle guide *Stomoxys* to bite and instantly then after thrust away the biting flies with the purpose of suck the blood at the biting site. Thus, the sucking flies boost the menace of mechanical transmission by *Stomoxys*. The mouthparts of sucking flies contaminate with *T. evansi* and then fly become the potential source of transmission of *T. evansi*. In a few cases, Reduviid bugs also found as a mechanical vector of *T. evansi*. The iatrogenic transmission by use of contaminated surgical instruments and use of contaminated needle in mass vaccination is also reported. Transmission from dam to calf during licking with parasitized secretions is also reported. *T. evansi* can also be transmitted through per os when carnivores take infected offal. That time parasite enters in circulation of carnivores by altered oral mucosa. Vampire bats (*Desmodus rotundus*) act as a true reservoir of *T. evansi*. Vampire bats suck the blood of infected host and become contaminated. The *T. evansi* multiply in bats and they die. Few bats survive and maintain chronic infection and act as a source of transmission of *T. evansi*.

## Origin

*T. evansi* was described by Griffith Evans, from the blood of Indian camels. *T. evansi* is thought to be derived from *T. brucei brucei* and transmitted cyclically by tsetse flies. The loss of maxicircles of kinetoplastic mitochondrial DNA in *T. brucei brucei* converts it into *T. evansi*. This evolution not only develops *T. evansi* but also diminishes its dependency on *Glossina* (Tse tse fly) for cyclical transmission.

## Geographical Distribution

*T. evansi* originated in Africa and started to spread eastwards towards Arabian peninsula, including Saudi Arabia, Oman, the United Arab Emirates, Jordan, Israel, Lebanon, Syria, Iraq, and Turkey, and even with one occasional record in Bulgaria; it is present from Iran to Kazakhstan as well as in Afghanistan and Pakistan and India. Now *T. evansi* also found in China, Mongolia, Russia, Bhutan, Nepal, Myanmar, Laos, Vietnam, Cambodia, Thailand, Malaysia, the Philippines, and Indonesia. The presence of *T. evansi* was suspected in Papua New Guinea and Australia. The extension of *T. evansi* toward the West is Latin America, Pantanal, Brazil, Bolivia, Venezuela, Guyana, Colombia and Mexico.

## Epidemiology

The epidemiology of a surra depends on the characteristics of a pathogen, its hosts, reservoir, and vectors and their environment and interrelations. In Asian subcontinent, the geographical distribution of *T. evansi* is spreading in large areas in India, China, and Russia. Horses, dogs, buffaloes, cattle, pigs and deer are the most susceptible species in Southeast Asia. In Asia, *T. evansi* mainly affects buffaloes and horses and acts as a reservoir of parasites. The disease is prevalent in animals challenged after hemorrhagic septicaemia vaccines. The Asian bovines show more pathogenicity than African and American strains. In India, *T. evansi* infection is everywhere in cattle, buffaloes, camels, donkeys, dogs, and horses.

## Economic Impact

There is a piece of limited information on the impact of trypanosomosis among livestock. It causes high mortality and reproductive losses in animals. The low calving performance, abortion and infertility impacts negatively on animals. The death of animals during their most productive phase reduces their life expectancy and has a major impact on farmers. Financial losses due to trypanosomosis can be avoided by implementing an effective control strategy. Diminazene aceturate is suggested as the most economical drug for treatment. The use of prophylactic drugs is also helpful to reduce the adverse economic impact of trypanosomosis in animals.

## Zoonotic Importance of *T. evansi*

The host range of *T. evansi* is various species of mammals except man. The propagation of *T. evansi* in man is inhibited by trypanolytic factor present in normal human serum. The trypanolytic factor is capable of killing Trypanosoma in human blood. The sub fractional studies revealed that a component, apolipoprotein L-1 (ApoL-1) is responsible for inhibition of *T. evansi* in human blood. A human case of trypanosomosis caused by *T. evansi* was reported from the Chandrapur district of Maharashtra, India in 2005. The study revealed that frameshift mutations in both Apo L-1 alleles in the case led to an unexpected termination of protein translation by internal stop codons, which resulted in a total absence of Apo L-1. Due to this, the protection is lost by human cases against *T. evansi* and the infection develops. A serological screening of humans near the first case by CATT/*T. evansi* showed up to 22.7% seropositivity. The trypanosomes were not detected in these persons during blood examinations. The reason was suggested that the human population is frequently exposed to *T. evansi* and killed Apo L-1.

## Clinical Signs

The general clinical signs of *T. evansi* are fever, anaemia, loss of appetite and weight, loss of body condition and productivity and nervous signs. The abortion, cachexia, and death is also reported in some cases. The intensity of clinical signs may vary from unapparent to lethal, depending on the host species and geographical location of the disease. Trypanosomosis by *T. evansi* is a disease of camelids and equines so, the typical clinical signs appear in these animals. In dairy animals especially cattle and buffaloes, *T. evansi* infection a mild, chronic or asymptomatic clinical signs are observed in Africa and Latin America. But in India and Mauritius, the clinical signs and pathogenic effect are recorded with very high mortality of 90%. Chronic infection of *T. evansi* infection in these areas results in anaemia, weight loss, production losses, and reduction in draught power, which can lead to totally wasted animals. Clinical signs include fever, anaemia, abortion, reduced body weight and irregular oestrous cycle and death of animal is reported in acute cases of infection. The clinical signs in buffaloes are fever, stiffness, conjunctivitis, emaciation, oedema of legs, inappetence, dyspnea, anaemia, recumbency, diarrhoea, abortion, and death. Sometimes nervous signs are also reported because of meningoencephalitis.

## Diagnosis

The definitive diagnosis involves various laboratory methods to demonstrate the parasites and serological tools to detect the specific antibodies of *Trypanosoma*. The primary biological sample is blood for the detection of *T. evansi*. However, other biological samples like cerebrospinal fluid (in the nervous form of trypanosomosis), joint fluid, or lymph node fluid can also be used. The different diagnostic methods for trypanosomosis are-

***Direct fresh mount of blood:*** A fresh drop of blood with anticoagulant is taken on a clean glass slide and examined microscopically in low magnification. The movement of trypanosomes is observed in positive cases. Trypanosome species show a peculiar type of movement. For example, *T. evansi* shows a jerky kind of movement.

***Hematocrit Centrifuge Technique (HCT)*****:** It is an enrichment method. In this suspected blood with anticoagulant is centrifuged and a smear is prepared using the upper layer of blood. The smear is stained and examined for trypanosomes. This method is helpful to detect 100–200 trypanosomes/mL of blood.

***Dark ground Buffy Coat Method (BCM)*****:** It is also an enrichment method in which a buffy coat is examined in a dark field microscope. Briefly, blood is taken in a microcapillary or quantitate buffy coat tube coated internally with acridine orange and then centrifuged at 1000 rpm for 5 minutes. The tube is examined in UV microscope or dark field microscope. The sensitivity of this method is almost equal to HCT and can detect 100–200 trypanosomes/mL of blood.

***Animal inoculation Method***: This method helps to detect subclinical infection. Briefly, 0.5 ml of suspected blood is inoculated intra-peritoneal in the laboratory rodent. After 3-5 days a smear is prepared by taking blood by cutting off the tail tip of the laboratory rodent. In positive cases, parasites are found in the blood smear. This method can detect parasitemia of 20– 50 parasites/mL of blood.

***Molecular Method***: DNA of *T. evansi* can be amplified using PCR with several specific primers. PCR is generally used to improve the sensitivity of the detection of trypanosomes. In this method, first DNA is isolated from suspected blood by standard protocol and then DNA is amplified by using specific primer. The study revealed that the Phenol-Chloroform method of DNA isolation and TBR primers for DNA amplification is the most sensitive for detecting *T. evansi*. This method can detect 5–10 trypanosomes/mL of blood.

***Serological tests***: Several serological tests can be performed to detect *T. evansi* in animals. They can be used to investigate prevalence or incidence studies at herd, seasonal or interannual variations follow-up and control method assessment. Agglutination test, double immune diffusion, complement fixation test, card agglutination and ELISA are a few of them. The most common methods are the Card Agglutination Test for *T. evansi* (CATT/*T. evansi*) and the ELISA *T. evansi*. CATT is worked on to detect immunoglobulin M and, therefore, early infections can be detected. Whereas ELISA is generally used to detect immunoglobulin G, therefore it is helpful to detect established infections. These tests are complementary to each other and can work well together. ELISA *T. evansi* is reasonably robust, regardless of the host species and provides the same range of sensitivity and specificity (90–95%) in the various host species including dairy animals. The sensitivity of CATT *T. evansi* varies from host to host. CATT shows very low sensitivity of approximately 12%in cattle.

***Chemical tests***: These tests detect alteration in serum protein in trypanosomosis. The alteration may also be possible in other diseases. So, these tests are non-specific and less reliable. However, these tests can be used for tentative diagnosis in field conditions. Among mercuric chloride test, formal gel test, thymol turbidity test, stilbamidine test and jone nitric acid test stilbamidine test is usable in bovines to detect trypanosomosis. In this test, approximately 2.0 ml of 10% solution of stilbamidine is added in a drop of suspected serum. The coagulation formed and the coagulum settled down in 30 seconds and dissolved in 5 to 10 minutes in positive cases.

## Treatment

***Chemical Control***: The two types of drugs are available for control of *T. evansi*. First one is the "curative drugs" used for treatment and having a short-term effect. The other one is a combination of "curative/preventive drugs" used for chemoprophylaxis. The curative/preventive drugs not only kill parasites but also prevent new infections due to the presence of a sustainable curative dose in the blood serum of animals. The commonly used drugs for trypanosomosis are-

1. **Diminazene aceturate (DA):** DA is an aromatic diamidine compound used for the treatment of *Babesia* and trypanosome infection in bovines and other ruminants. The curative recommended dose of DA is 7mg/kg body weight via intramuscular injection in ruminants. The withdrawal period for DA is 21 days for meat and 3 days for milk. The previous dose of 3.5 mg/kg bw of DA for treatment is now considered as underdosing that leads to the selection of chemoresistant strains of *Trypanosoma*. It is a preferred drug at a dose of 7mg/kg bw by intramuscular injection in cattle and buffaloes. In the case of high parasitaemia is an initial administration of 3.5mg/kg bw DA to reduce the parasitaemia and a second administration of 7mg/kg bw can be given after 5 days to kill all the trypanosomes.

2. **Isometamidium chloride (IMC):** IMC is a homidium chloride or bromide under family phenanthridine. Homidium chloride or bromide compounds are the DNA intercalating agents having mutagenic action. Because of highly toxic nature at gene level their use in the field is not recommended. The curative and preventive dose of IMC is 0.5mg/kg bw and 1mg/kg bw respectively for trypanosomosis in ruminants. This can be administered via intramuscular or subcutaneous route. The withdrawal period for IMC in cattle is 23 days. The IMC retains in the blood for up to 4-5 months after injection. So, a safe withdrawal period is suggested around 3 months at the dose rate of 0.5mg/kg and 6 months at the dose rate of 1mg/kg bw. The very high withdrawal periods make IMC disappointingly adapted to beef or dairy cattle. In case of ineffectiveness of treatment, the use of IMC is recommended at a dose of 0.5 mg/kg in cattle.

   **Note:** An alternate use of DA and IMC makes a "sanative pair," means that once resistance develops to one of the compound, the other compound should be used to control the infection.

3. **Melarsomine dihydrochloride (Cymelarsan):** It is an organic arsenical chemotherapeutic agent and the latest drug first time use for trypanosomosis in camel. Now the dose rate of cymelarsan is 0.5mg/kg bw in cattle and 0.75mg/kg bw in buffaloes. The animals treated with cymelarsan may show nervous signs.

4. **Suramin:** It is a ureic component used in horses and camels only by intravenous injection against *T. evansi.* Now the drug is no longer used.

5. **Quinapyramine:** The compound is an aminoquinaldine derivative. Two compounds Quinapyramine sulphate and quinapyramine chloride are used for trypanosomosis for curative and prophylactic purposes respectively in horses and camels. Triquin is a combination of quinapyramine sulphate and quinapyramine chloride that can be used as a curative/preventive drug against *T. evansi*. The dose rate of triquin is 8mg/kg bw and the route of administration is sub-cutaneous. The drug is quite effective in chemoprophylactic effect against trypanosomosis. It gives prophylactic effect for 4 months. Quinapyramine may induce cross-resistance to both DA and IMC and is thus not recommended in cattle.

## Control

The control of vector-transmitted disease classically can be divided into pathogen control and vector control. There is no vaccine available and a limited chance of developing of vaccine against *T. evansi* shortly disease control is chiefly based on the use of trypanocides and vector control.

1. ***Trypanocides*:** The trypanocides for control of *T. evansi* has been described in treatment section.

2. ***Vector Control*:** It is quite effective strategy to control of trypanosomosis in animals. Control of tabanid vectors is a difficult task because of the fly diversity in an area, high mobility and prolificacy. The larvae of tabanids are generally spread over a wide area and different species colonize at various landscapes. So, the insecticide sprays is not suitable for long periods. The insecticide spray is an effective strategy for 2-3 years; after that, the tabanid reappears. Tabanid control in large open areas is unsuccessful because tabanids move in from the surrounding areas to fill the ecological gap. So, the tabanid control by insecticide is considered as costly, unsatisfactory and unsustainable. *Stomoxys* is another vector for transmission of trypanosomosis in animals. *Stomoxys* proliferate and develop within the livestock rearing area and are thus closely related

to the farming systems. *Stomoxys* population can be controlled by management practices.

Different traps are used to control of vector. Among them, the most effective traps for the control of mechanical vectors are the Nzi trap and the Vavoua trap. The Nzi trap is used to catch the large tabanid flies and *Stomoxys*, while the Vavoua trap is used to catch small tabanid species, such as *Chrysops*. Use of insecticides like deltamehrin on the body of animals can also be used for fly control. However, the effectiveness is relatively short which makes control system costly. Use of smoke released by slow fire is an alternative and traditional method for fly control but limited to small areas. The smoke also reduces the food intake in animals.

Mosquito nets can also be used to protect animals from flies. The insecticide impregnation of nets increases the effectiveness of mosquito nets. The "Japanese net" is used to catch the vampire bats in Latin America. Then the cached bats are coated with an anticoagulant (e.g. chlorophacinone) with excipient and released. Once the bat returns to its colony, it spreads the anticoagulant because of excipient to the colony by licking and contact. This process kills the bats of the colony within a few days.

## Immune Evasion Mechanism by *Trypanosoma evansi*

The Trypanosomes are covered with the glycoprotein surface which is antigenic in nature and provokes the antibody responses in the host. This causes opsonization and lysis of the trypanosomes. Despite the effective immune effector mechanism, trypanosomes have an effective ability to evade the immune response by changing the antigenic composition of their glycoprotein surface coat. The term is called "antigenic variation". The trypanosomes alter the chemical composition of their glycoprotein coat and now, display a different antigenic surface called variant surface glycoprotein (VSG). This causes the trypanosomes unaffected by the developed antibody. The trypanosomes having this new variant antigen multiply to produce a second wave of parasitaemia. Again the host produces a new antibody against new variant surface glycoprotein, but again the glycoprotein coat is altered by trypanosomes so that a third wave of parasitaemia arises. This process of antigenic variation is associated with waves and remissions of parasitaemias, often at weekly intervals, and may continue for several months. The animal may die due to parasitemia. The repeated change of the glycoprotein coat is mediated by a loosely ordered sequential expression of an undefined number of genes. These genes code the different glycoprotein coats in trypanosomes. So, the trypanosomes in circulation become a mixture of different antigenic types, those expressing a different genetic repertoire. This is the reason behind why animals susceptible to reinfection immediately even after it treated successfully for trypanosomosis. The vaccine development is difficult against trypanosomosis due to the above mentioned reason.

## References


Abou El-Naga, T., Barghash, S., Mohammed, A., Ashour, A. and Salama, M.S., 2012. Evaluation of (Rotat 1. 2-PCR) assays for identifying Egyptian Trypanosoma evansi DNA. Acta Parasitologica Globalis, 3(1), pp.1-6.

Adrian, M.S., Sani, R.A., Hassan, L. and Wong, M.T., 2010. Outbreaks of trypanosomiasis and the seroprevalence of T. evansi in a deer breeding centre in Perak, Malaysia. Tropical Animal Health and Production, 42, pp.145-150.

Bhaskara Rao, T., Balarama Raju, P., Hararama Das, J. and Hafeez, M., 1995. Some observations on an outbreak of surra in circus tigers.

Bullard, W., Kieft, R., Capewell, P., Veitch, N.J., Macleod, A. and Hajduk, S., 2012. Haptoglobin-hemoglobin receptor independent killing of African trypanosomes by human serum and trypanosome lytic factors. Virulence, 3(1), pp.72-76.

Coura, J.R. and Borges-Pereira, J., 2010. Chagas disease: 100 years after its discovery. A systemic review. Acta tropica, 115(1-2), pp.5-13.

Cuisance D, Politzar H, Merot P, Tamboura I. Les lâchers de mâles irradiés dans la campagne de lutte intégrée contre les glossines dans la zone pastorale de Sidéradougou (Burkina Faso).

Dargantes, A.P., Mercado, R.T., Dobson, R.J. and Reid, S.A., 2009. Estimating the impact of Trypanosoma evansi infection (surra) on buffalo population dynamics in southern Philippines using data from cross-sectional surveys. International journal for parasitology, 39(10), pp.1109-1114.

Dargantes, A.P., Mercado, R.T., Dobson, R.J. and Reid, S.A., 2009. Estimating the impact of Trypanosoma evansi infection (surra) on buffalo population dynamics in southern Philippines using data from cross-sectional surveys. International journal for parasitology, 39(10), pp.1109-1114.

Davila, A.M. and SILVA, R.A.M., 2000. Animal trypanosomiasis in South America: current status, partnership, and information technology. Annals of the New York Academy of Sciences, 916(1), pp.199-212.

de Oliveira Lima, A.N., da Silva Santos, S., Herrera, H.M., Gama, C., Cupolillo, E., Jansen, A.M. and Fernandes, O., 2008. Trypanosoma evansi: molecular homogeneity as inferred by phenetical analysis of ribosomal internal transcribed spacers DNA of an eclectic parasite. Experimental parasitology, 118(3), pp.402-407.

Desquesnes, M., Biteau-Coroller, F., Bouyer, J., Dia, M.L. and Foil, L., 2009. Development of a mathematical model for mechanical transmission of trypanosomes and other pathogens of cattle transmitted by tabanids. International Journal for Parasitology, 39(3), pp.333-346.

Desquesnes, M., Holzmuller, P., Lai, D.H., Dargantes, A., Lun, Z.R. and Jittaplapong, S., 2013. Trypanosoma evansi and surra: a review and perspectives on origin, history, distribution, taxonomy, morphology, hosts, and pathogenic effects. BioMed research international, 2013(1), p.194176.

Dia, M.L., Desquesnes, M., Elsen, P., Lancelot, R. and Acapovi, G., 2004. Evaluation of a new trap for tabanids and stomoxyines. Bulletin de la Societe Royale Belge d'Entomologie, 140, pp.72-81.

Dia, M.L. and Desquesnes, M., 2007. Infections ecpérimentales de bovins par Trypanosoma evansi pathogénicité et efficacité du traitement au Cymelarsan.

Dobson, R.J., Dargantes, A.P., Mercado, R.T. and Reid, S.A., 2009. Models for Trypanosoma evansi (surra), its control and economic impact on small-hold livestock owners in the Philippines. International journal for parasitology, 39(10), pp.1115-1123.

Dávila, A.M.R., Herrera, H.M., Schlebinger, T., Souza, S.S. and Traub-Cseko, Y.M., 2003. Using PCR for unraveling the cryptic epizootiology of livestock trypanosomosis in the Pantanal, Brazil. Veterinary parasitology, 117(1-2), pp.1-13.

Foil, L.D., Adams, W.V., McManus, J.M. and Issel, C.J., 1987. Bloodmeal residues on mouthparts of Tabanus fuscicostatus (Diptera: Tabanidae) and the potential for mechanical transmission of pathogens. Journal of medical entomology, 24(6), pp.613-616.

García, H., García, M.E., Pérez, G., Bethencourt, A., Zerpa, E., Pérez, H. and Mendoza-León, A., 2006. Trypanosomiasis in Venezuelan water buffaloes: association of packed-cell volumes with seroprevalence and current trypanosome infection. Annals of Tropical Medicine & Parasitology, 100(4), pp.297-305.

García, H., García, M.E., Pérez, G., Bethencourt, A., Zerpa, E., Pérez, H. and Mendoza-León, A., 2006. Trypanosomiasis in Venezuelan water buffaloes: association of packed-cell volumes with seroprevalence and current trypanosome infection. Annals of Tropical Medicine & Parasitology, 100(4), pp.297-305.

Gardiner, P.R. and Mahmoud, M.M., 1992. Salivarian trypanosomes causing disease in livestock outside sub-Saharan Africa.

Gibson, W., 2007. Resolution of the species problem in African trypanosomes. International journal for parasitology, 37(8-9), pp.829-838.

Gill, B.S., 1977. Trypanosomes and trypanosomiases of Indian livestock.

Gutierrez, C., Corbera, J.A., Juste, M.C., Doreste, F. and Morales, I., 2005. An outbreak of abortions and high neonatal mortality associated with Trypanosoma evansi infection in dromedary camels in the Canary Islands. Veterinary Parasitology, 130(1-2), pp.163-168.

Gutierrez, C., Desquesnes, M., Touratier, L. and Büscher, P., 2010. Trypanosoma evansi: recent outbreaks in Europe. Veterinary Parasitology, 174(1-2), pp.26-29.

Haridy, F.M., El-Metwally, M.T., Khalil, H.H. and Morsy, T.A., 2011. Trypanosoma evansi in dromedary camel: with a case report of zoonosis in greater Cairo, Egypt. Journal of the Egyptian Society of Parasitology, 41(1), pp.65-76.

Hasan, M.U., Muhammad, G., Gutierrez, C., Iqbal, Z., Shakoor, A. and Jabbar, A., 2006. Prevalence of Trypanosoma evansi infection in equines and camels in the Punjab region, Pakistan. Annals of the New York Academy of Sciences, 1081(1), pp.322-324.

Hoare, C.A., 1972. Trypanosomes of mammals: A zoological monograph.

Jensen, R.E., Simpson, L. and Englund, P.T., 2008. What happens when Trypanosoma brucei leaves Africa. Trends in Parasitology, 24(10), pp.428-431.

Jittapalapong, S., Pinyopanuwat, N., Inpankaew, T., Sangvaranond, A., Phasuk, C., Chimnoi, W., Kengradomkij, C., Kamyingkird, K., Sarataphan, N., Desquesnes, M. and Arunvipas, P., 2009. Prevalence of Trypanosoma evansi infection causing abortion in dairy cows in central Thailand. Agriculture and Natural Resources, 43(5), pp.53-57.

Kumar, R., Kumar, S., Khurana, S.K. and Yadav, S.C., 2013. Development of an antibody-ELISA for seroprevalence of Trypanosoma evansi in equids of North and North-western regions of India. Veterinary parasitology, 196(3-4), pp.251-257.

Kurup, S.P. and Tewari, A.K., 2012. Induction of protective immune response in mice by a DNA vaccine encoding Trypanosoma evansi beta tubulin gene. Veterinary Parasitology, 187(1-2), pp.9-16.

Lamborn, W.A., 1936. The experimental Transmission to Man of Treponema pertenue by the Fly Musca sorbens Wd.

Laveissière, C. and Grebaut, P., 1990. The trapping of tsetse flies (Diptera: Glossinidae). Improvement of a model: the Vavoua trap. Tropical medicine and parasitology: Official organ of Deutsche Tropenmedizinische Gesellschaft and of Deutsche Gesellschaft fur Technische Zusammenarbeit (GTZ), 41(2), pp.185-192.

Lun, Z.R., Min, Z.P., Huang, D., Liang, J.X., Yang, X.F. and Huang, Y.T., 1991. Cymelarsan in the treatment of buffaloes naturally infected with Trypanosoma evansi in South China. Acta Tropica, 49(3), pp.233-236.

Mandal, M., Laha, R. and Sasmal, N.K., 2008. First report of establishment of Trypanosoma evansi infection in pigeon nestlings (Columba livia). Journal of Parasitology, 94(6), pp.1428-1429.

Manz, P., 1985. Studies on the transmission of Trypanosoma evansi (Steel, 1885) via local tabanids (Diptera, Tabanidae) and South American reduviids (Hemiptera, Reduviidae).

Masiga, D.K., Smyth, A.J., Hayes, P., Bromidge, T.J. and Gibson, W.C., 1992. Sensitive detection of trypanosomes in tsetse flies by DNA amplification. International journal for parasitology, 22(7), pp.909-918.

Mdachi, R.E., Murilla, G.A., Omukuba, J.N. and Cagnolati, V., 1995. Disposition of diminazene aceturate (Berenil®) in trypanosome-infected pregnant and lactating cows. Veterinary Parasitology, 58(3), pp.215-225.

Mekata, H., Konnai, S., Mingala, C.N., Abes, N.S., Gutierrez, C.A., Dargantes, A.P., Witola, W.H., Inoue, N., Onuma, M., Murata, S. and Ohashi, K., 2012. Kinetics of regulatory dendritic cells in inflammatory responses during Trypanosoma evansi infection. Parasite Immunology, 34(6), pp.318-329.

Mihok, S., 2002. The development of a multipurpose trap (the Nzi) for tsetse and other biting flies. Bulletin of Entomological Research, 92(5), pp.385-403.

Milocco, C., Kamyingkird, K., Desquesnes, M., Jittapalapong, S., Herbreteau, V., Chaval, Y., Douangboupha, B. and Morand, S., 2013. Molecular demonstration of Trypanosoma evansi and Trypanosoma lewisi DNA in wild rodents from Cambodia, Lao PDR and Thailand. Transboundary and Emerging Diseases, 60(1), pp.17-26.

Muhammad, G., Saqib, M., Sajid, M.S. and Naureen, A., 2007. Trypanosoma evansi infections in Himalayan black bears (Selenarctos thibetanus). Journal of Zoo and wildlife Medicine, 38(1), pp.97-100.

Murray, M., Murray, P.K. and McIntyre, W.I.M., 1977. An improved parasitological technique for the diagnosis of African trypanosomiasis. Transactions of the Royal Society of Tropical Medicine and Hygiene, 71(4), pp.325-326.

Njiru, Z.K., Constantine, C.C., Masiga, D.K., Reid, S.A., Thompson, R.C.A. and Gibson, W.C., 2006. Characterization of Trypanosoma evansi type B. Infection, Genetics and Evolution, 6(4), pp.292-300.

Oliveira, C.B., Da Silva, A.S., Souza, V.C., Costa, M.M., Jaques, J.A., Leal, D.B., Lopes, S.T. and Monteiro, S.G., 2012. NTPDase activity in lymphocytes of rats infected by Trypanosoma evansi. Parasitology, 139(2), pp.232-236.

Payne, R.C., Sukanto, I.P., Partoutomo, S., Jones, T.W., Luckins, A.G. and Boid, R., 1994. Efficacy of Cymelarsan in Friesian Holstein calves infected with Trypanosoma evansi. Tropical animal health and production, 26(4), pp.219-226.

Pruvot, M., Kamyingkird, K., Desquesnes, M., Sarataphan, N. and Jittapalapong, S., 2010. A comparison of six primer sets for detection of Trypanosoma evansi by polymerase chain reaction in rodents and Thai livestock. Veterinary parasitology, 171(3-4), pp.185-193.

Radwanska, M., Guirnalda, P., De Trez, C., Ryffel, B., Black, S. and Magez, S., 2008. Trypanosomiasis-induced B cell apoptosis results in loss of protective anti-parasite antibody responses and abolishment of vaccine-induced memory responses. PLoS pathogens, 4(5), p.e1000078.

Raina, A.K., Kumar, R., Sridhar, V.R. and Singh, R.P., 1985. Oral transmission of Trypanosoma evansi infection in dogs and mice. Veterinary Parasitology, 18(1), pp.67-69.

Reid, S.A. and Copeman, D.B., 2000. Surveys in Papua New Guinea to detect the presence of Trypanosoma evansi infection. Australian Veterinary Journal, 78(12), pp.843-845.

Russel, D. and Sambrook, J., 2001. Molecular cloning: a laboratory manual. New.

Seidl, A.F., Moraes, A.S. and Silva, R.A.M.S., 2001. Trypanosoma evansi control and horse mortality in the Brazilian Pantanal. Memorias do Instituto Oswaldo Cruz, 96, pp.599-602.

Sharma, D.K., Saxena, V.K. and Agrawal, R.D., 2000. Haematological changes in experimental trypanosomiasis in Barbari goats. Small Ruminant Research, 38(2), pp.145-149.

Sharma, G. and Juyal, P.D., 2007. Trypanosomosis in a German shepherd dog–A case report. Journal of Veterinary Parasitology, 21(1), pp.81-82.

Silva, A.S.D., Ceolin, L.V., Oliveira, C.B., Monteiro, S.G. and Doyle, R.L., 2007. Oral infection by Trypanosoma evansi in rats and mice. Ciencia Rural, 37, pp.897-900.

Silva, R.A.M.S., Egüez, A., Morales, G., Eulert, E., Montenegro, A., Ybañez, R., Seidl, A., Rivera Dávila, A.M. and Ramirez, L., 1998. Bovine trypanosomiasis in Bolivian and Brazilian lowlands. Memórias do Instituto Oswaldo Cruz, 93, pp.29-32.

Singh, N., Pathak, K.M.L. and Kumar, R., 2004. A comparative evaluation of parasitological, serological and DNA amplification methods for diagnosis of natural Trypanosoma evansi infection in camels. Veterinary Parasitology, 126(4), pp.365-373.

Singla, L.D., Juyal, P.D. and Sharma, N.S., 2010. Immune responses to haemorrhagic septicaemia (HS) vaccination in Trypanosoma evansi infected buffalo-calves. Tropical Animal Health and Production, 42, pp.589-595.

Sinha, P.K., Mukherjee, G.S., Das, M.S. and Lahiri, R.K., 1971. Outbreak of tripanosomiasis evansi amongst tigers and jaguars in the Zoological Garden, Calcutta.

Sudarto, M.W., Tabel, H. and Hainies, D.M., 1990. Immunohistochemical demonstration of Trypanosoma evansi in tissues of experimentally infected rats and a naturally infected water buffalo (Bubalus bubalis). The Journal of parasitology, pp.162-167.

Tager-Kagan P, Itard J, Clair M. Essai de l'efficacité du Cymelarsan (ND) sur Trypanosoma evansi chez le dromadaire.

Tarello, W., 2005. Trypanosoma evansi infection in three cats.

Tejero, F., Roschman, G., Perrone, C. and Aso, P.M., 2008. Trypanosoma evansi: A quantitative approach to the understanding of the morphometry-hematology relationship throughout experimental murine infections. The journal of protozoology research, 18(1), pp.34-47.

Toro M, Leon E, Lopez R, Pallota F, Garcia JA, Ruiz A. Effect of isometamidium on infections by Trypanosoma vivax and T. evansi in experimentally-infected animals. Veterinary Parasitology. 1983 Aug 1;13(1):35-43.

Tuntasuvan, D., Jarabrum, W., Viseshakul, N., Mohkaew, K., Borisutsuwan, S., Theeraphan, A. and Kongkanjana, N., 2003. Chemotherapy of surra in horses and mules with diminazene aceturate. Veterinary Parasitology, 110(3-4), pp.227-233.

Upadhye, S.V. and Dhoot, V.M., 2000. Trypanosomiasis in a tiger (Panthera tigris).

Vanhollebeke, B. and Pays, E., 2010. The trypanolytic factor of human serum: many ways to enter the parasite, a single way to kill. Molecular microbiology, 76(4), pp.806-814.

Veer, V., Parashar, B.D. and Prakash, S., 2002. Tabanid and muscoid haematophagous flies, vectors of trypanosomiasis or surra disease in wild animals and livestock in Nandankanan Biological Park, Bhubaneswar (Orissa, India). Current science, 82(5), pp.500-503.

Vergne, T., Kamyinkird, K., Desquesnes, M. and Jittapalapong, S., 2011. Attempted transmission of Trypanosoma evansi to rats and mice by direct ingestion of contaminated blood and via engorged ticks. Acta Protozoologica, 50(2).

World Health Organization, 2005. A new form of human trypanosomiasis in India: description of the first human case in the world caused by Trypanosoma evansi. Weekly Epidemiological Record= Relevé épidémiologique hebdomadaire, 80(07), pp.62-63.

# 3

# Theileria

***Jitendra Tiwari[1], Amit Kumar Jaiswal[1] and Mukesh K Srivastava[2]***

*[1]Department of Veterinary Parasitology, U. P. Pandit Deen Dayal Upadhyaya Pashu Chikitsa Vigyan Vishwavidyalaya Evam Go Anusandhan Sansthan (DUVASU), Mathura, Uttar Pradesh*
*[2]Department of Veterinary Medicine, U. P. Pandit Deen Dayal Upadhyaya Pashu Chikitsa Vigyan Vishwavidyalaya Evam Go Anusandhan Sansthan (DUVASU), Mathura, Uttar Pradesh*

Theileriosis is a tick-borne protozoan disease that affects a wide range of domestic and wild animals, particularly cattle. While multiple species of *Theileria* exist, *Theileria parva* and *Theileria annulata* are the most important pathogens in terms of their impact on domestic cattle. This disease is transmitted by ixodid ticks and has a significant impact on cattle populations in tropical and subtropical regions. Theileriosis poses a substantial threat to livestock productivity, affecting economic stability in many countries, especially those that rely heavily on agriculture and cattle farming.

The disease has two primary forms: East Coast fever (ECF), caused by *T. parva*, which predominantly affects cattle in eastern, central, and southern Africa; and tropical theileriosis, caused by *T. annulata*, which affects cattle across northern Africa, the Middle East, and parts of Asia. Both diseases are highly pathogenic and, if left untreated, can lead to high morbidity and mortality rates, significantly impacting livestock production.

Theileriosis, particularly East Coast fever, was first identified in southern Africa at the end of the 19th century, where cattle herds experienced devastating outbreaks of a disease characterized by high fever, lymphadenopathy, and high mortality. It was eventually linked to the bite of ticks, and the causative organism was identified as *Theileria parva*, named after Arnold Theiler, the Swiss veterinarian who contributed significantly to the study of this disease. Over time, tropical theileriosis caused by *T. annulata* was discovered in the Mediterranean basin, northern Africa, and parts of Asia, and it soon became clear that this disease, while distinct from East Coast fever, posed a similar threat to cattle health.

Initially, cattle owners and farmers struggled to manage the disease due to a lack of knowledge about its transmission and pathology. The disease spread rapidly in regions where tick populations flourished, leading to severe losses in cattle production. Control efforts were limited to managing ticks through traditional methods, which were often ineffective. The development of acaricides (chemical compounds used to kill ticks) and vaccines marked significant progress in controlling theileriosis, though challenges in eradication remain due to the parasite's complex life cycle and its ability to evade the host's immune defenses.

Theileriosis poses significant challenges to livestock health in many parts of Africa, Asia, and Southern Europe, where the disease is endemic. Affected animals may show severe symptoms, including fever, anemia, lymphadenopathy, and in severe cases, death. Without effective control measures, theileriosis can lead to substantial economic losses due to decreased productivity, high mortality rates, and the cost of treatment and prevention.

The complex relationship between the parasite, its tick vector, and the mammalian host makes theileriosis a difficult disease to control. Various strategies, including tick control, chemotherapy, and vaccination, have been implemented with varying degrees of success. This assignment provides an in-depth examination of theileriosis, focusing on its causative agents, epidemiology, clinical manifestations, and control measures.

### Causative Agents

Theileriosis is caused by several species of the protozoan parasite *Theileria*, which belongs to the phylum Apicomplexa. The two most important species affecting cattle are:

- ***Theileria parva:*** This species is responsible for East Coast fever (ECF), a highly fatal disease prevalent in eastern and southern Africa. It primarily affects cattle but can also infect other ruminants.
- ***Theileria annulata:*** This species causes tropical theileriosis, which is found in parts of North Africa, the Middle East, and Asia. It is transmitted by ticks of the genus *Hyalomma* and can lead to significant morbidity and mortality in affected cattle.

*Theileria* parasites are intracellular, and their life cycle involves both a mammalian host and a tick vector. The parasites invade and proliferate within leukocytes (white blood cells) and erythrocytes (red blood cells), leading to significant immune suppression and pathology in the host.

## Life Cycle

The life cycle of the *Theileria* parasite is a complex, multi-stage process that involves two primary hosts: a tick vector and a mammalian host, typically cattle. This parasite has a unique ability to infect and proliferate within host cells, particularly leukocytes and erythrocytes, which leads to significant immunosuppression and damage to the host.

The life cycle of *Theileria* involves both asexual and sexual reproduction stages, with critical transformations taking place within the tick vector and the mammalian host.

### • Infection of the Bovine Host: Sporozoite Invasion

The life cycle of *Theileria* begins when an infected ixodid tick, such as *Rhipicephalus appendiculatus* (for *T. parva*) or *Hyalomma* spp. (for *T. annulata*), feeds on a susceptible bovine host. During feeding, the tick injects sporozoites, the infective stage of the *Theileria* parasite, into the bloodstream of the animal through its saliva.

• The sporozoites are motile and quickly seek out and invade host leukocytes, particularly macrophages, monocytes, and lymphocytes. This stage of the parasite's life cycle is critical, as the successful invasion of leukocytes sets the stage for the asexual reproduction of the parasite. Inside the leukocyte, the sporozoite transforms into a schizont, the first replicative form of the parasite in the mammalian host. The transformation of sporozoites into schizonts is rapid and marks the beginning of the proliferative stage of the parasite within the host's immune cells.

### • Schizogony: Intracellular Proliferation of Schizonts

Once inside the host leukocytes, *Theileria* schizonts undergo a process called schizogony, a form of asexual reproduction. This stage is characterized by the rapid multiplication of the parasite within the host cell. The schizonts divide and cause the infected leukocytes to undergo clonal expansion, leading to an uncontrolled proliferation of the leukocytes.

The schizonts essentially hijack the host cell's regulatory machinery, transforming the infected leukocytes into proliferating tumor-like cells. This uncontrolled division of leukocytes leads to the enlargement of lymphoid organs, such as lymph nodes and the spleen, causing clinical symptoms such as lymphadenopathy (swollen lymph nodes). As the infected leukocytes proliferate, they disseminate throughout the host's body, spreading the infection to various tissues and organs.

During schizogony, the host immune system is severely compromised, as the unchecked proliferation of infected leukocytes disturbs normal immune function. The leukocyte expansion also facilitates the spread of the parasite throughout the body, allowing it to invade additional cells and tissues. This systemic infection is responsible for many of the severe clinical manifestations of theileriosis, such as fever, immunosuppression, and respiratory distress.

**• Merozoite Formation and Erythrocyte Invasion**

As the schizonts continue to proliferate within leukocytes, they eventually differentiate into merozoites, which are the next stage in the parasite's life cycle. This differentiation marks the transition from the leukocytic phase to the erythrocytic phase of the infection. Once formed, the merozoites are released from the infected leukocytes and enter the bloodstream, where they seek out and invade erythrocytes.

The invasion of erythrocytes by merozoites is another critical stage in the life cycle of *Theileria*, as this phase is responsible for the development of piroplasms, the form of the parasite that is transmissible to ticks. Inside the erythrocytes, the merozoites differentiate into small, ring-shaped forms known as piroplasms. In *T. annulata* these piroplasms are non-proliferative within the RBCs but remain in the bloodstream, whereas division of piroplasms has been reported in case of *T. parva*. These piroplasms are available for uptake by feeding ticks.

The erythrocytic phase of the infection is associated with anemia and jaundice in the host, as the destruction of red blood cells leads to a significant decrease in the oxygen-carrying capacity of the blood. In severe cases, this can result in life-threatening anemia, particularly in young or immunocompromised animals. The erythrocytic phase also plays a critical role in the transmission of the disease, as the piroplasms are necessary for the continuation of the parasite's life cycle in the tick vector.

**• Transmission Back to the Tick: Ingestion of Piroplasms**

The next stage in the life cycle of *Theileria* occurs when an uninfected tick feeds on an infected bovine host. During the tick's blood meal, it ingests RBCs containing piroplasms. Once inside the tick, the piroplasms are released from the erythrocytes and undergo sexual reproduction within the tick's gut, forming zygotes.

The zygotes then migrate to the tick's salivary glands, where they differentiate into sporozoites. This process of sexual reproduction and subsequent sporozoite formation is crucial for the parasite's development within the tick and for the transmission of the infection to new hosts. The tick serves as a biological vector for the disease, harboring the sporozoites until its next feeding event, when it will transmit the parasite to another bovine host.

It is important to note that different tick species serve as vectors for different *Theileria* species. For example, *Rhipicephalus appendiculatus* is the primary vector for *T. parva*, while *Hyalomma anatolicum* is responsible for the transmission of *T. annulata*. The biology and ecology of the tick vectors play a significant role in the epidemiology of theileriosis, as the distribution of the disease is closely linked to the presence and abundance of the tick populations in a given area.

**• Sporozoite Development and Transmission to New Hosts**

Once the sporozoites have developed in the tick's salivary glands, they are ready to be transmitted to a new host during the tick's next blood meal. When the tick feeds on a susceptible bovine host, it injects the sporozoites into the host's bloodstream, initiating the cycle once again.

## 4. Epidemiology of Theileriosis

The epidemiology of theileriosis is shaped by a combination of environmental, vector, and host factors. The disease remains a significant threat to cattle populations in tropical and subtropical regions, where it leads to heavy economic and social burdens. Effective control requires a comprehensive understanding of local conditions, vector ecology, and host susceptibility, as well as the implementation of integrated management practices that target both the tick vectors and the *Theileria* parasite itself.

**• Geographical Distribution**

Theileriosis is endemic in many parts of Africa, Asia, and the Middle East, with distinct geographic distributions based on the species of *Theileria* and their tick vectors.

**East Coast Fever (*T. parva*):** East Coast fever is primarily found in sub-Saharan Africa, stretching from Sudan in the north to Mozambique in the south and from the Indian Ocean coast to parts of central Africa. The primary vector of *T. parva* is the brown ear tick (*Rhipicephalus appendiculatus*), which thrives in areas with a warm, humid climate and bushy vegetation. East Coast fever is particularly prevalent in eastern and southern Africa, affecting countries such as Kenya, Uganda, Tanzania, Zambia, and Malawi.

**Tropical Theileriosis (*T. annulata*):** Tropical theileriosis is found in North Africa, the Middle East, southern Europe, and large parts of Asia, including

India, Pakistan, and China. The primary vector for *T. annulata* is the *Hyalomma* tick, which is well-adapted to drier and more arid climates. *Hyalomma* ticks are common in regions with semi-arid conditions, making tropical theileriosis a major concern in areas with harsh, dry climates such as northern Africa and western Asia. Countries like Iran, Iraq, Turkey, and parts of India and Pakistan experience high disease incidence.

**• Tick Vectors and Environmental Factors**

Theileriosis is a tick-borne disease, and the presence, abundance, and distribution of ticks are key determinants of its epidemiology. *Theileria* parasites are transmitted by specific tick species, and the seasonal activity of these ticks is heavily influenced by environmental factors such as temperature, humidity, and vegetation.

**Tick Species and Activity:** The brown ear tick, *R. appendiculatus* thrives in warm and moist environments with dense vegetation, while *Hyalomma* ticks are more prevalent in arid and semi-arid regions with sparse vegetation. The activity of ticks, and therefore the transmission of *Theileria* parasites, tends to peak during the rainy season when humidity is high and vegetation is abundant. Tick populations decline during dry seasons or in very hot or cold conditions, which can temporarily reduce disease transmission.

**• Host Susceptibility and Breed Factors**

Different cattle breeds have varying levels of susceptibility to *Theileria* infection, which influences disease prevalence and severity.

**Indigenous vs. Exotic Breeds**: Indigenous cattle breeds, such as *Bos indicus* and East African Zebu, often exhibit a certain level of resistance or tolerance to *Theileria* infection. These breeds have co-evolved with the disease and the tick vectors in their native environments, allowing them to develop some degree of immunity. On the other hand, exotic or high-yielding breeds like Holstein-Friesian, Jersey, and crossbred cattle are highly susceptible to the disease. These breeds are often introduced into endemic regions for improved milk production, but their lack of resistance to *Theileria* makes them more vulnerable to severe illness and death.

**Age and Immunity:** Young cattle, particularly those less than one year old, are more susceptible to the disease than adult cattle. Calves born in endemic areas may acquire some passive immunity through maternal antibodies, but this protection is short-lived. Immunity in cattle that survive natural infection or are vaccinated is long-lasting, making them less likely to develop severe disease upon subsequent tick infestations.After undergoing schizogony, the schizonts differentiate into merozoites, which are released from the leukocytes. These merozoites then invade erythrocytes, initiating the erythrocytic phase of the infection. Inside the red blood cells, merozoites develop into piroplasms, which are the forms that can be transmitted to ticks during their next feeding.

The destruction of erythrocytes during this phase contributes to the development of anemia, a common clinical feature of severe theileriosis. The anemia is exacerbated by the immune-mediated destruction of infected and uninfected erythrocytes, leading to a further decrease in the host's oxygen-carrying capacity. This can result in jaundice, weakness, and, in severe cases, death.

## Immune Response to Theileriosis

The immune response to *Theileria* infection is complex, as the parasite manipulates the host's immune system in several ways. The immune system is forced to confront an intracellular pathogen that can hide within immune cells, making it challenging to mount an effective defense. Nevertheless, both innate and adaptive immune responses play crucial roles in controlling the infection.

The initial immune response to *Theileria* infection is mediated by the innate immune system, particularly through the activation of macrophages and dendritic cells. These cells detect the presence of the parasite via pattern recognition receptors (PRRs), which recognize pathogen-associated molecular patterns (PAMPs) expressed by *Theileria*. This triggers the release of pro-inflammatory cytokines such as TNF-α, IL-1, and IL-6, which are crucial for activating other immune cells and initiating the inflammatory response.

However, as *Theileria* infects and hijacks macrophages and other leukocytes, it can subvert this immune defense mechanism. By transforming infected cells into proliferating, immortalized cells, the parasite impairs the host's innate immune response. The uncontrolled proliferation of infected cells leads to widespread tissue damage and immunosuppression, creating an environment in which the parasite can thrive.

The adaptive immune response is critical for controlling and eventually clearing *Theileria* infection. Both humoral (antibody-mediated) and cellular (T cell-mediated) immunity are involved in the response to the parasite. Cytotoxic T lymphocytes play a vital role in the control of this infection. CTLs recognize and kill infected leukocytes, particularly those harboring schizonts, via the presentation of parasite antigens on the surface of infected cells. However, due to the immunosuppressive effects of the disease, CTL responses are often delayed or weakened, allowing the parasite to persist in the host.

Antibodies produced by B cells can target extracellular stages of the parasite, such as sporozoites and merozoites, limiting their ability to invade new cells. In particular, neutralizing antibodies can prevent sporozoites from invading leukocytes and may also target piroplasms in the erythrocytic phase of the infection. However, since *Theileria* spends most of its life cycle within host cells, humoral immunity alone is not sufficient to clear the infection.

## 6. Clinical Manifestations in Cattle

The clinical signs of theileriosis vary depending on the species of *Theileria* involved, the level of parasitemia, and the immune status of the host. Common clinical manifestations include:

### *A. Acute Clinical Signs*

The acute form of theileriosis, particularly associated with *T. parva*, is characterized by severe clinical signs that can lead to high mortality rates, especially in susceptible cattle breeds. Key clinical manifestations include:

- **Fever**: A sudden onset of high fever (up to 41°C or 105.8°F) is one of the earliest and most prominent signs. The fever is often intermittent and can persist for several days.
- **Lymphadenopathy**: Swelling of lymph nodes is a common finding. The superficial lymph nodes, particularly those in the cervical and submandibular regions, become enlarged and can be palpated easily.
- **Anemia**: Due to the destruction of RBCs caused by both the parasite and the immune response, affected cattle often show signs of anemia. This can manifest as pallor of the mucous membranes, weakness, and lethargy.
- **Jaundice**: The destruction of RBCs can lead to elevated bilirubin levels, resulting in jaundice. Affected animals may exhibit yellowing of the sclera of the eyes and other mucosal surfaces.
- **Respiratory Distress**: As the disease progresses, some cattle may exhibit signs of respiratory distress due to severe anemia or secondary infections.
- **Coughing and Nasal Discharge**: These can also be observed in some cases, particularly if there is secondary respiratory involvement.

### *B. Sub-acute and Chronic Forms*

In some cases, especially in indigenous breeds that exhibit a degree of resistance, clinical manifestations may be less severe, resulting in subacute or chronic forms of the disease. These include:

- **Weight Loss**: Progressive weight loss due to reduced feed intake, chronic disease, and metabolic demands may be noted over time.
- **Reduced Milk Production**: In lactating cows, there is often a noticeable decline in milk yield as a consequence of the disease.
- **Chronic Lethargy**: Animals may appear lethargic and less active than normal, often preferring to isolate themselves from the herd.
- **Persistent Fever**: Low-grade fever can persist in chronic cases, leading to a state of unthriftiness.

### *C. Neurological Signs*

In severe cases, particularly with *T. parva*, neurological signs may develop due to the involvement of the central nervous system. This can manifest as:

- **Ataxia**: Lack of coordination and unsteady gait may be observed.
- **Depression**: Affected cattle may appear depressed, with decreased responsiveness to external stimuli.

### *D. Mortality Rates*

The mortality rates associated with theileriosis can be significantly high, especially in naive populations of susceptible cattle. Without prompt and effective treatment, death may occur within two to three weeks after the onset of clinical signs.

## 7. Diagnosis of Theileriosis

Accurate and timely diagnosis of theileriosis is essential for effective management and control of the disease, particularly in endemic regions where it poses a significant threat to cattle health and productivity. The diagnosis of theileriosis relies on a combination of clinical evaluation, history of exposure to tick vectors, and laboratory tests.

### *A. Clinical Assessment*

The initial step in diagnosing theileriosis involves a thorough clinical examination of the affected animal.

- **Clinical Signs**: Observations of symptoms such as fever, lymphadenopathy, anemia, jaundice, and respiratory distress are critical. The presence of these clinical signs, especially in regions where theileriosis is endemic, raises suspicion of the disease.

- **History of Tick Exposure**: Information regarding the animal's history, including exposure to ticks and previous instances of theileriosis in the herd, can assist in the diagnosis. Cattle in tick-infested areas, particularly those with high populations of *Rhipicephalus appendiculatus* or *Hyalomma* ticks, are at greater risk.

### *B. Laboratory Diagnostics*

While clinical assessment can provide valuable clues, definitive diagnosis typically requires laboratory testing. Several diagnostic methods are commonly employed:

- **Blood Smear Examination**: This is the most traditional method for diagnosing theileriosis. A blood sample is taken from the suspect animal and stained with Giemsa or Wright's stain. Under a microscope, the presence of *Theileria* parasites, particularly in the form of schizonts in leukocytes or piroplasms in erythrocytes, can be identified. This method is quick and cost-effective, but sensitivity can be limited, especially in chronic cases where parasite levels may be low.
- **Serological Tests**: Enzyme-linked immunosorbent assays (ELISA) and indirect immunofluorescence assays (IFA) can detect antibodies against *Theileria* species. These tests are useful for identifying exposure to the parasite, even in cases where the blood smear is negative. However, serological tests may not distinguish between active infection and past exposure.
- **Polymerase Chain Reaction (PCR)**: Molecular techniques, particularly PCR, have gained popularity for the diagnosis of theileriosis due to their high sensitivity and specificity. PCR can detect the genetic material of the *Theileria* parasite in blood samples, allowing for the identification of the specific species involved. This method is particularly advantageous in cases where low parasite loads may evade detection by microscopy.

### *C. Differential Diagnosis*

Given that the clinical signs of theileriosis can overlap with other diseases affecting cattle, differential diagnosis is crucial. Conditions such as bovine babesiosis, anaplasmosis, and other infectious diseases should be considered. Laboratory tests and clinical history can help differentiate these diseases based on specific symptoms, response to treatment, and laboratory findings.

## 8. Treatment and Control

The management of theileriosis in cattle involves both treatment strategies for infected animals and comprehensive control measures aimed at reducing the prevalence of the disease in the herd and the environment. Given the serious economic implications associated with this disease, effective treatment and prevention are essential. The treatment of theileriosis focuses on alleviating clinical signs, managing symptoms, and eradicating the parasite from the host. The following are key components of treatment:

**Antiparasitic Medications**: The primary treatment for theileriosis involves the use of single dose of Buparvaquone @ 2.5 mg/kg b. wt. intramuscularly. Treatment is efficacious when administered during the initial phases of clinical illness. Treatment is less efficacious in advanced stages characterized by significant loss of lymphoid and haematopoietic tissues. Resistance to buparvaquone has also been documented in *T. annulata*.

- **Supportive Care**: In addition to antiparasitic treatment, supportive care is critical for improving recovery rates. Administering intravenous fluids can help combat dehydration and support the animal's overall health, particularly in cases of severe anemia or dehydration.
- **Anti-inflammatory and Antibiotic Therapy**: Non-steroidal anti-inflammatory drugs can be administered to reduce fever and inflammation. Antibiotics may also be used to prevent or treat secondary bacterial infections, which can complicate the disease.
- **Monitoring and Follow-up**: Continuous monitoring of the animal's condition and response to treatment is essential. Follow-up blood tests may be conducted to evaluate the effectiveness of the treatment and to check for any residual parasitemia.

### Control Measures

Effective control of theileriosis relies on a combination of strategies aimed at reducing the exposure of cattle to *Theileria*-infected ticks and managing the overall health of the herd:

- **Tick Control**: Implementing effective tick control measures is the cornerstone of preventing theileriosis. Strategies include:
    - **Chemical Control**: Regular application of acaricides to reduce tick populations on cattle and in their environment can significantly decrease the risk of transmission. It is important to follow recommended dosages and application schedules to avoid resistance development.

- **Pasture Management**: Keeping pastures clean and managing vegetation can help minimize tick habitats. Rotating grazing areas may also reduce tick exposure.

- **Vaccination**: Rakshavac-T is intended for the prophylaxis of Theileriosis induced by *Theileria annulata.* Rakshavac-T comprises live schizonts cultivated in lymphoblast cell culture, which have been attenuated through extended in-vitro passage. Vaccinated cattle can endure the infection for a duration of three years.

- **Herd Management Practices**: Maintaining overall herd health is crucial in reducing the impact of theileriosis. This includes:
  - **Regular Health Monitoring**: Routine veterinary check-ups and health monitoring can help identify and treat infections early.
  - **Isolation of New Animals**: New animals should be quarantined and tested for diseases, including theileriosis, before introduction into the herd.

The economic impact of theileriosis on the livestock industry is profound. Infected animals exhibit decreased productivity, including reduced milk yield, weight loss, and reproductive failure. The cost of treating affected animals and implementing tick control measures adds to the financial burden on farmers. Moreover, high mortality rates in cattle herds can lead to devastating losses, particularly for smallholder farmers in endemic regions. In regions heavily affected by the disease, theileriosis can lead to significant trade restrictions, as countries may impose barriers to livestock imports from endemic areas due to the risk of disease transmission.

The control of theileriosis faces several challenges, including the emergence of acaricide-resistant tick populations, vaccine development issues, and the difficulty of maintaining effective control programs in resource-limited settings. Future research should focus on:

- Developing more effective and sustainable tick control strategies.
- Improving vaccines against both *Theileria* parasites and tick vectors.
- Exploring genetic resistance to *Theileria* in cattle breeds.
- Strengthening veterinary infrastructure and farmer education programs in endemic regions.

Theileriosis remains a major threat to livestock health in many parts of the world, with significant economic and public health implications. While progress has been made in controlling the disease, particularly through vaccination and tick control, challenges persist. A coordinated, multi-faceted approach that integrates veterinary science, farmer education, and sustainable tick control practices is essential for reducing the burden of theileriosis and improving livestock productivity.

## References

Abdela, N. and Bekele, T., 2016. Bovine theileriosis and its control: a review. Advances in Biological Research, 10(4), pp.200-212.

Agina, O.A., Shaari, M.R., Isa, N.M.M., Ajat, M., Zamri-Saad, M. and Hamzah, H., 2020. Clinical pathology, immunopathology and advanced vaccine technology in bovine theileriosis: A review. Pathogens, 9(9), p.697.

Kahn C.M. Ed. (2005). – Merck Veterinary Manual, 9th Edition. Merck & Co. Inc. and Merial Ltd. Whitehouse. Station, NJ: Merck. • Spickler, Anna Rovid.

Soulsby, E.J.L., 1982. Helminths, arthropods and protozoa of domesticated animals (No. 7th edition, 809pp).

Theileriosis. Retrieved from World Organisation for Animal Health (2024). – Manual of Diagnostic Tests and Vaccines for Terrestrial Animals. OIE, Paris.

# 4

# Babesia

*Vivek Agrawal[1], Nidhi S Choudhary[2], Mukesh Shakya[1], Supriya Shukla[3], Girraj Goyal[4], and Binita Kumari Singh[1]*

[1]*Department of Veterinary Parasitology, College of Veterinary Science and A.H., Mhow, NDVSU, Jabalpur-453446, Madhya Pradesh, India*
[2]*Department of Veterinary Medicine, College of Veterinary Science and A. H., Mhow, NDVSU, Jabalpur-453446, Madhya Pradesh, India*
[3]*Department of Veterinary Pathology, College of Veterinary Science & A.H. Mhow, NDVSU, Jabalpur-453446, Madhya Pradesh, India*
[4]*Department of Poultry Science, College of Veterinary Science and Animal Husbandry, NDVSU, Jabalpur- 482001 (M.P.)*

Bovine babesiosis is a significant febrile disease, primarily affecting cattle and buffalo, transmitted by ticks. The disease is marked by the rapid proliferation of parasites within the bloodstream, leading to the extensive destruction of red blood cells. This results in a cascade of clinical symptoms, including anemia, jaundice, hemoglobinuria, and splenomegaly, with the potential for severe cases to culminate in death. The acute form of bovine babesiosis is particularly severe, often characterized by these pronounced symptoms, which can lead to rapid deterioration in the affected animals. Babesiosis is not merely an acute illness but can also persist as a chronic infection. Chronic bovine babesiosis is typified by ongoing anemia and varying degrees of weight loss, reflecting the enduring impact of the parasite within the host. Economically, this disease poses a formidable challenge, especially in regions where cattle are most susceptible. Since the first description of *Babesia bovis* by Victor Babes in Romania in 1888, numerous distinct species have been identified, each contributing to the global burden of this disease (Hunfeld et al., 2008). The impact of bovine babesiosis on livestock improvement efforts in endemic regions is profound. The introduction of susceptible, naive animals into these areas often leads to significant losses, as these animals are highly vulnerable to the disease. The repercussions of an outbreak extend beyond immediate health concerns, encompassing broader economic losses such as reduced milk production, increased treatment costs, decreased fertility in bulls, and even abortion in pregnant cows. A strong correlation exists between the prevalence of bovine babesiosis and the distribution of its vector ticks, particularly in tropical and subtropical regions. The transmission of *Babesia* spp. is exclusively through tick bites, where the ticks, having fed on infected animals, transfer the parasite to healthy hosts during subsequent feedings. The lifecycle of these ticks further exacerbates the situation, as they can pass the infection to their offspring through their eggs, ensuring the persistence of the disease across generations (Taylor et al., 2004). Bovine babesiosis is a global concern, with its presence noted in nearly every region where cattle are raised. In tropical countries like India, the climatic conditions are particularly conducive to the proliferation of ticks, which infest a wide variety of hosts, from small mammals like mice to large domestic and wild animals such as elephants. Ticks are also found on birds and reptiles, further complicating control efforts. Their ability to infest such a diverse range of hosts makes ticks notoriously difficult to eradicate from the environment. The persistent presence of ticks on domesticated animals remains a significant concern, posing ongoing challenges to the control and prevention of bovine babesiosis.

## 1. Etiology

Bovine babesiosis is caused by protozoan parasites of the genus *Babesia*, within the order Piroplasmida and phylum Apicomplexa. The primary species responsible for this disease are *Babesia bovis*, *Babesia bigemina*, *Babesia divergens*, and *Babesia major*. Of these, *B. bovis* and *B. bigemina* are the most prevalent and significant, particularly in tropical and subtropical regions, with *B. bovis* being the more pathogenic strain (Homer et al., 2000). These parasites are a major concern in these regions due to their severe impact on cattle health and the livestock industry.

## 2. Host

Cattle are the primary hosts for bovine babesiosis, though other ungulates such as water buffalo, African buffalo, and various wild species can also be infected. However, these alternative hosts are generally not significant in the transmission of the disease. Native cattle breeds, particularly *Bos indicus*, exhibit a high level of resistance to babesiosis, whereas crossbred cattle are much more vulnerable, necessitating the implementation of control measures to prevent outbreaks (Montenegro-James, 1992). Age is a critical factor in susceptibility; while younger animals are more resistant to infection, clinical disease incidence tends to increase as cattle age. Newborn calves, especially those born to immune mothers, benefit from innate immunity that protects them from babesiosis for up to six months (Agrawal et al., 2020). In contrast, infection is rare in cattle older than five years. The transmission dynamics also vary between *Babesia* species: *Babesia bigemina* primarily infects cattle under one year of age, while *Babesia bovis* is more frequently observed in cattle older than two years. Immune-compromised and stressed animals, particularly those that are pregnant or in poor condition, are the most susceptible to severe infection. This underscores the need for vigilant management practices in susceptible populations to mitigate the impact of bovine babesiosis on livestock health and productivity.

## 3. Life Cycle

In animals, protozoa responsible for babesiosis are present in the bloodstream only during the active stages of infection. The transmission of this disease is primarily facilitated by ticks, which act as natural vectors by harboring the parasite during a portion of its life cycle. Notably, *Rhipicephalus* species, formerly known as *Boophilus* spp., including *Boophilus microplus*, are capable of carrying both *Babesia bovis* and *Babesia bigemina* for a significant part of their life cycle. *Boophilus annulatus* and *B. microplus* are the main tick species involved in the transmission of babesiosis (Riek, 1964). *Boophilus* spp. and *Babesia* spp. exhibit a specific parasitic relationship with their hosts, targeting only erythrocytes in vertebrates. Once a sporozoite from *Babesia* penetrates the erythrocyte membrane, it begins its maturation process, resulting in the formation of two merozoites. The developmental stages of *Babesia*, known as trophozoites, progress as the parasite multiplies within the erythrocyte. During blood transfer from the host to the tick vector's midgut, gametocytes undergo a division process, producing two populations of ray bodies. These ray bodies continue to multiply and eventually fuse to form a zygote.

The zygote then invades the tick's digestive cells, where it undergoes further development into kinetes. These motile, club-shaped kinetes escape into the tick's hemolymph, from where they disseminate to various cell types and tissues, including the oocytes. The secondary schizogony process repeats in the oocytes, leading to transovarial transmission during the tick's larval stage. This transmission mechanism ensures that the parasite is passed on to the next generation of ticks( Fig. 01).

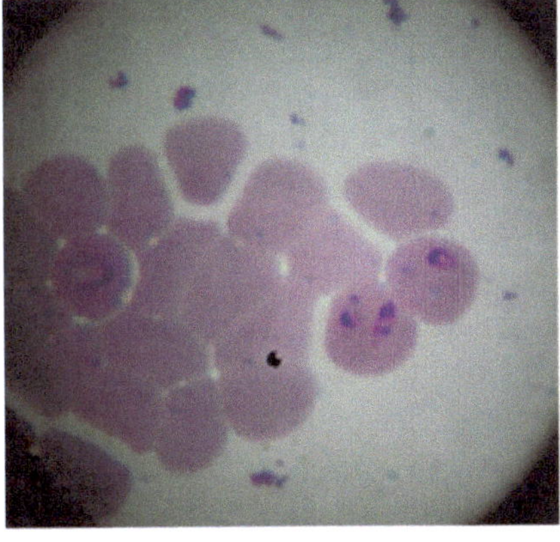

**Fig. 4.1:** *Babesia bigemina* in thin blood smear stained with giemsa stain

The infected tick's development typically halts before the vertebrate host is infected. This crucial stage occurs when the kinetes penetrate the tick's salivary glands and transform into sporozoites, ready to be transmitted to a new host. Besides tick bites, infection can also be spread through contaminated needles and surgical instruments, highlighting the importance of sterile practices in veterinary care to prevent iatrogenic transmission of babesiosis.

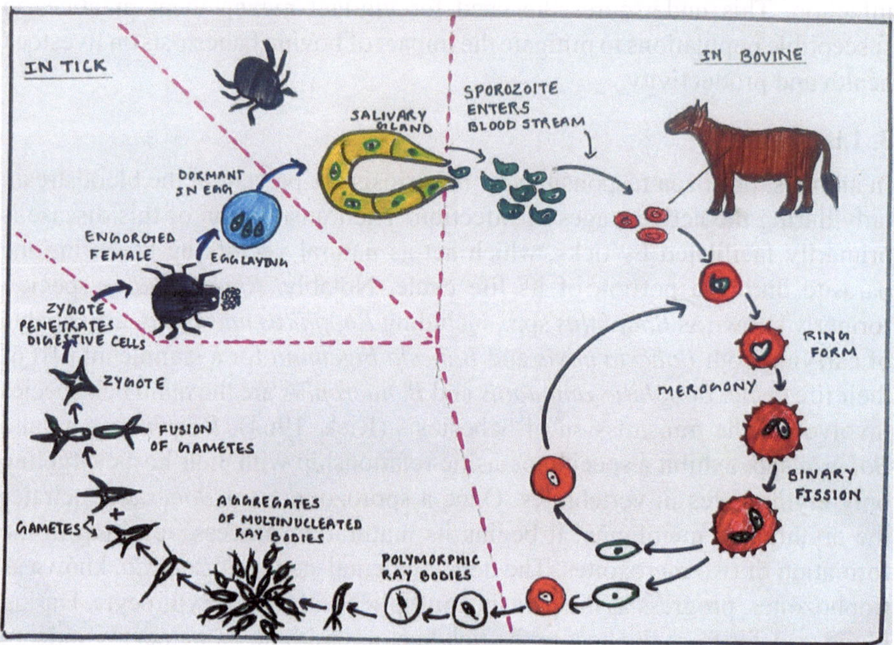

Fig. 4.2: General lifecycle of *Babesia*

## 4. Pathogenesis

In the pathogenesis of *Babesia bovis* infections, the immune response plays a crucial role, with cytokines and other pharmacologically active substances being central to this process. However, the overproduction of these mediators can exacerbate the disease, leading to a range of severe clinical manifestations. These include vasodilation, hypotension, increased capillary permeability, edema, vascular collapse, coagulation disorders, endothelial damage, and circulatory stasis. The severity of these outcomes is closely tied to the timing and quantity of cytokine production. The most devastating pathophysiological effects often occur in the brain and lungs, even though microcirculatory stasis, caused by the aggregation of infected erythrocytes in capillary beds, is a significant feature. This can lead to cerebral babesiosis and respiratory distress syndrome, conditions characterized by neutrophil infiltration, increased vascular permeability, and edema (Agrawal et al., 2023).

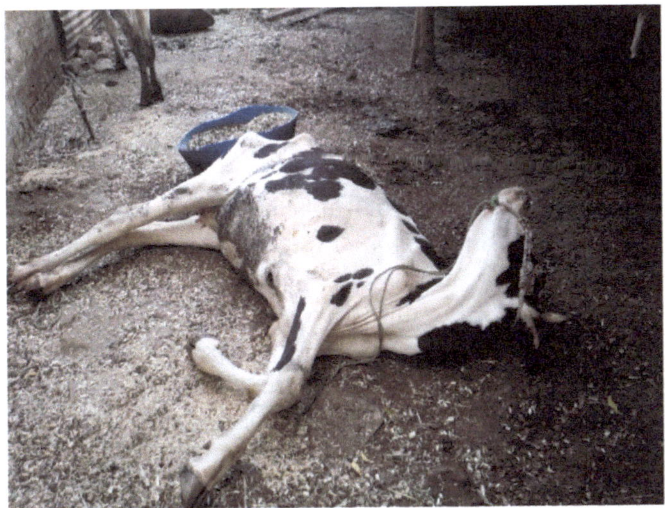

**Fig. 4.3:** Cerebral babesiosis unveiling the neurological signs

Progressive hemolytic anemia is another significant consequence of *B. bovis* infections, particularly in chronic cases. While this anemia may not be prominent during the acute phase, it contributes significantly to disease progression in prolonged infections. The acute phase typically lasts three to seven days, during which fever (exceeding 40°C) is a persistent symptom, often appearing several days before other clinical signs. These signs include inappetence, depression, increased respiratory rate, weakness, and reluctance to move. The condition, known as "redwater" in some regions, frequently presents with hemoglobinuria. Anemia and jaundice become more pronounced in prolonged cases. In severe instances, the disease progresses to muscle atrophy, tremors, recumbency, and eventually coma. Fever associated with *B. bovis* infections can also lead to abortion in pregnant cattle and reduced fertility in bulls for up to six to eight weeks.

Cerebral babesiosis, a severe complication of *B. bovis* infection, presents with a wide range of neurological symptoms and is almost always fatal. Post-mortem examinations often reveal an enlarged, soft spleen, a swollen liver, a distended gall bladder filled with thick, granular bile, congested and dark-colored kidneys, and generalized anemia and jaundice. Pulmonary edema may be present, and other organs may show signs of congestion or petechial hemorrhages. The brain's grey matter may exhibit a pink hue. Hemoglobinuria, a hallmark of acute cases, may be absent in subacute or chronic cases. Clinical pathology primarily focuses on macrocytic and hypochromic hemolytic anemia. In non-fatal cases, recovery can be prolonged, taking several weeks, but it is usually complete. Subacute infections are less overt and may be challenging to diagnose. Calves infected before nine months of age typically exhibit subclinical rather than full-blown infections. Recovered animals can remain asymptomatic carriers for extended periods, with the duration of infection varying by breed.

*Babesia bigemina* infections, while similar in some respects, differ significantly in their pathogenesis. The primary pathological feature is rapid and often massive intravascular hemolysis. Unlike *B. bovis* infections, *B. bigemina* does not typically cause coagulation disorders, cytoadherence, or hypotension. Instead, the pathogenic effects are more directly related to the destruction of erythrocytes. Hemoglobinuria is more consistent and appears earlier in the course of *B. bigemina* infections, while fever is less prominent. Cattle affected by *B. bigemina* acutely are generally less severely impacted than those with *B. bovis* infections. In cases that do not result in death, cerebral involvement is absent, and recovery is usually swift and complete. However, in some instances, the disease can progress rapidly, leading to sudden and severe anemia, jaundice, and death with little or no warning.

Recovered animals from *B. bigemina* infections remain infectious to ticks for four to seven weeks and carry the parasite for only a few months. The carrier state in *B. bigemina* is thus shorter and less persistent compared to *B. bovis*, which has implications for disease control and management strategies in endemic areas.

## 5. Endemic Stability

Endemic stability, a concept crucial to understanding the dynamics of babesiosis, refers to a state where the interaction between the host, pathogen, vector, and environment is balanced, leading to infrequent or negligible occurrences of clinical disease. This equilibrium is largely influenced by the development of innate immunity in calves. Initially, calves possess passive immunity acquired from maternal antibodies, which typically lasts for about two months before waning. However, when calves are exposed to babesiosis within the first six to nine months, they rarely show clinical symptoms and develop long-lasting immunity.

Endemic stability is maintained when a significant proportion of the calf population is exposed to *Babesia* infection early in life. If at least 75% of calves are exposed to *B. bovis* by the time they are six to nine months old, the incidence of disease would be minimal, achieving a state of natural endemic stability. The transmission dynamics of *B. bovis* play a critical role in this process. Despite the fact that a single infected tick is sufficient to transmit *B.*

*bovis*, the overall infection rate among ticks tends to be low, resulting in a slow transmission rate to cattle. For instance, a field study in Australia revealed that only 0.04% of larval ticks were infected with *B. bovis* in paddocks where *Bos taurus* cattle were present, with even lower percentages observed in areas stocked with *Bos indicus* cattle (Mahoney et al., 1981).

In contrast, *B. bigemina* has a higher infection rate in ticks, with studies reporting an infection rate of 0.23%. Consequently, the transmission rates for *B. bigemina* are generally higher, and endemic stability for this species is more easily established compared to *B. bovis*. This difference in transmission dynamics means that regions where both *Babesia* species coexist are more likely to achieve endemic stability with *B. bigemina*.

Mathematical models have become essential tools in predicting endemic stability within cattle herds. Early models estimating infection rates in calves based on serological data provided valuable insights into the status of *Babesia bovis* infections. Although these models showed efficacy with certain cattle breeds, their accuracy across other breeds proved less reliable. To enhance prediction capabilities, a more advanced model was developed, which refines the approach by quantifying incidence risk using age-specific seroprevalence data. This updated model translates the data into a comprehensive herd framework, estimating the distribution of animals across various disease severity levels by age and sex. The model's application has been pivotal in forecasting the potential impact of *Babesia* species on large-scale cattle operations and in performing cost-benefit analyses of management strategies. Such predictive tools are invaluable for implementing effective control measures and maintaining herd stability in endemic regions .

## 6. Immunity

The immune response in cattle to infections caused by *Babesia bovis* and *Babesia bigemina* is a complex interplay between innate and acquired immunity. Understanding this immune response is essential to controlling the spread and impact of bovine babesiosis, a disease with significant economic and public health implications.

### i. Innate Immunity

Innate immunity is the first line of defense against babesiosis, shaped by several factors, including host-parasite specificity, genetic predisposition, and age. The spleen plays a pivotal role in this defense, particularly in its ability to suppress parasitemia in cattle. Research has demonstrated that splenectomized cattle, or those without a spleen, exhibit significantly higher levels of parasitemia when infected with *Babesia*, underscoring the spleen's critical role in immune response. Interestingly, cattle breeds display varying levels of susceptibility to *B. bovis* and *B. bigemina* infections. Despite extensive research, the genetic factors that influence this susceptibility remain elusive. Age is also a crucial determinant, with young calves showing a robust innate immune response, potentially due to the early induction of cytokines like IL-12 and IFN-c, along with the expression of inducible nitric oxide synthase (iNOS) in the spleen. This immune response diminishes with age, highlighting the unique resilience of young calves (Zintl et al., 2005).

Activated monocytes, macrophages, and neutrophils are central to the innate immune response, producing antimicrobial compounds like reactive nitrogen intermediates (RNI) and reactive oxygen species (ROS) that combat the parasite. The production of nitric oxide (NO) by macrophages, triggered by cytokines such as IFN-c and TNF-a, has been shown to reduce *B. bovis* viability, emphasizing the importance of these immune cells in the battle against the parasite. Furthermore, oxidative bursts within phagocytes, resulting in the production of ROS, are crucial in the babesicidal activity against *B. bovis.*

### ii. Acquired Immunity

The acquired immune response to *Babesia* infection involves a sophisticated interplay of antibodies and T cells. Hyperimmune serum from repeatedly infected cattle, rich in IgG1 and IgG2 antibodies, has been shown to confer protection against *B. bovis*. These antibodies likely function as opsonins, enhancing phagocytosis rather than directly attacking the parasite. The role of T cells, particularly CD4+ helper T cells, is central to this response, with cytokines like IFN-c driving the activation of phagocytic cells and the production of antibodies by B cells. However, cross-species immunity between *B. bovis* and *B. bigemina* remains elusive. While *B. bigemina* offers some protection against *B. bovis*, the reverse is not true. Antibody-mediated immunity is species-specific, with homologous antibodies persisting longer after infection with *B. bovis* compared to *B. bigemina.*

### iii. Duration and Variability of Immunity

The duration of immunity following infection with *B. bovis* and *B. bigemina* varies significantly. Immunity to *B. bovis* can last for at least four years, while immunity to *B. bigemina* tends to wane after six months. Interestingly, the presence of detectable antibodies does not necessarily correlate with immunity, as some cattle can remain immune long after antibodies become undetectable. The persistence of *Babesia* infections is also influenced by antigenic variation, where the parasite changes its surface antigens to evade the host's immune system. This variation allows *Babesia* to maintain a latent infection in cattle, with periodic recrudescence of parasitemia. The ability of the parasite to adhere to endothelial cells, thereby avoiding splenic clearance, further complicates the immune response, allowing the parasite to persist despite apparent immunity. In conclusion, the immune response to bovine babesiosis is a dynamic and intricate process involving both innate and acquired mechanisms. While significant progress has been made in understanding these processes, challenges remain, particularly in the development of cross-species immunity and the management of antigenic variation. Understanding these mechanisms is crucial for developing effective control strategies against this economically significant disease.

## 7. Diagnosis and Validation of Bovine Babesiosis

Bovine babesiosis, a disease primarily transmitted by *Boophilus* ticks, manifests with a variety of clinical symptoms in cattle, including fever, anemia, jaundice, hemoglobinuria, and the characteristic appearance of an enlarged, dark, pulpy spleen. These symptoms are typically observed in cattle residing in enzootic regions where the presence of these ticks is prevalent. The accurate diagnosis of bovine babesiosis is critical for effective disease management and can be validated through multiple diagnostic methods, including microscopic examination, serologic testing, and transmission studies.

i. **Microscopic Examination and Blood Smears:** The initial step in diagnosing bovine babesiosis involves the microscopic examination of blood smears. It is recommended to prepare both thick and thin blood smears from live animals, ideally targeting capillaries from the ear or tail tip for sample collection (Homer et al., 2000). While jugular blood collected in EDTA is typically used for hematologic studies, acute and convalescent sera are required for serological testing. Additionally, during necropsy, smears from various organs—including the heart muscle, kidney, liver, lung, and brain—should be obtained, along with blood from a peripheral extremity. Blood and organ smears are invaluable for confirming the presence of tick fever, particularly when examining capillary blood from the tail tip. Organ smears, even from animals that have been deceased for up to 24 hours, can still be useful for diagnosis. During acute infections, *Babesia bigemina* can often be detected on thin blood smears stained with Giemsa (Fig. 02). Although thicker smears may increase the likelihood of identifying the organism, they can obscure the typical morphology, making identification more challenging.

ii. **Serological Testing and Antibody Detection:** For chronic infections, where the parasite may be present in very low numbers or even undetectable shortly after the acute phase, serological assays are the preferred method for diagnosis. These assays are designed to detect specific antibodies against *Babesia* species, providing a means to confirm a diagnosis and guide treatment decisions. The Indirect Fluorescent Antibody Technique (IFAT) and enzyme-linked immunosorbent assays (ELISA) are commonly employed in laboratory settings for this purpose. IFAT is used to identify antibodies specific to *Babesia bovis* and *Babesia bigemina*. In contrast, ELISA offers a more efficient approach for detecting antibodies across a large number of samples, making it an invaluable tool for both diagnostic and epidemiological studies. Specifically, the *Babesia bigemina* ELISA is a competitive assay that utilizes recombinant antigens to coat microtitre plates, thereby enhancing its accuracy. Meanwhile, the Babesia bovis ELISA relies on crude antigens from laboratory cultures.

iii. **Molecular Diagnostics and Emerging Techniques:** Advances in molecular diagnostics have led to the development of DNA probes capable of detecting extremely low parasitemias, such as those found in carrier animals. Although these techniques hold significant promise for the future, their practical application in routine diagnostics is still limited (Weiss, 1995). Additionally, infected ticks can be identified through haemolymph and egg smears, which provide another avenue for diagnosing babesiosis in chronically affected or carrier animals.

iv. **Transmission Studies and Histopathology:** In cases where the diagnosis is challenging due to the absence of hemoglobinuria or low parasitemias, transmission tests can be employed to confirm infection. This involves inoculating a fully susceptible animal, preferably a splenectomized cow, with 500 milliliters of blood from the suspected carrier and then monitoring for signs of infection. Histopathological examination further aids in diagnosis by revealing significant reductions in erythrocyte count, packed cell volume, and hemoglobin concentration, as well as increased bleeding tendencies and accelerated red blood cell sedimentation.

v. **Differential Diagnosis:** When diagnosing bovine babesiosis, it is crucial to consider other conditions that may present with similar clinical signs.

These include anaplasmosis, trypanosomiasis, theileriosis, leptospirosis, bacillary hemoglobinuria, post-parturient hemoglobinuria, enzootic bovine pyelonephritis, and chronic copper poisoning. In particular, cerebral babesiosis must be differentiated from other central nervous system disorders, such as rabies and plant toxicosis, to ensure accurate diagnosis and appropriate treatment (Ali and Marif, 2023). The diagnosis of bovine babesiosis requires a multifaceted approach that combines clinical observation, microscopic examination, serological testing, and, in some cases, molecular diagnostics and transmission studies. By employing these methods, veterinarians and researchers can accurately identify and manage this tick-borne disease, ultimately reducing its impact on cattle populations in enzootic regions. The ongoing development of more sophisticated diagnostic tools, such as DNA probes, holds the potential to further enhance the accuracy and efficiency of babesiosis diagnosis, paving the way for improved disease control and prevention strategies in the future

## 8. Treatment

Early treatment during the initial stages of infection significantly enhances the likelihood of success. However, if treatment is delayed, supportive therapies and blood transfusions may become necessary to save the animal. Smaller *Babesia* species typically exhibit higher resistance to chemotherapy. It is crucial to initiate therapy promptly, ideally before the onset of anemia, even if parasitemia is reduced. Care must be taken to avoid complete parasitemia clearance before sufficient antibodies are generated to confer long-term immunity.

A recommended treatment involves the administration of Imizol 12%—a subcutaneous injection at a dosage of 1 ml per 100 kg, equivalent to 1 mg/kg body weight of imidocarb dipropionate salt. For chemoprophylaxis, a higher dose of 3 mg/kg body weight (Imizol 12%—2.5 ml per 100 kg subcutaneously) can be effective in preventing clinical infection for up to two months. This allows a mild subclinical infection as the drug level decreases, eventually leading to premunition and immunity. However, it is important to note that Imizol administration can impair the animal's immunity to tick fever; hence, vaccination should be postponed for at least eight weeks post-treatment.

In the diagnosis process, thick smears, despite making it more challenging to discern unique morphology, increase the chances of detecting the causative organism. Given the low parasitemia in *B. bovis* infections, brain biopsies are particularly useful in enhancing the detection and diagnosis of the infection. Chronic infections are generally diagnosed through various serological tests that identify specific antibodies, as the organism either disappears or is present in extremely low levels shortly after the acute phase.

Serological testing, including the Indirect Fluorescent Antibody Technique (IFAT) and enzyme-linked immunosorbent assay (ELISA), is employed to confirm diagnoses and provide additional information. The *B. bovis* ELISA is used extensively as a diagnostic and epidemiological tool to detect antibodies in large sample sets. In this method, microtitre plates are coated with crude *B. bovis* antigen. The *B. bigemina* ELISA, a competitive assay, utilizes recombinant antigen-coated microtitre plates for improved accuracy.

It is essential to consider differential diagnoses, including anaplasmosis, trypanosomiasis, theileriosis, leptospirosis, bacillary haemoglobinuria, postparturient haemoglobinuria, enzootic bovine pyelonephritis, and chronic copper poisoning. The clinical manifestations of cerebral babesiosis must also be distinguished from other central nervous system conditions such as rabies and plant toxicosis (Fig. 03).

## 9. Prevention and Control

Effective prevention and control strategies are crucial in managing babesiosis. Modern control methods include the use of acaricides to prevent tick infestations, vaccination of susceptible livestock, administration of chemoprophylaxis, treatment of infected animals, regulation of livestock movement, and breeding cattle resistant to ticks. In endemic regions, management interventions are often unnecessary, as native cattle typically become infected as calves. To maintain an enzootically stable state, it is essential to expose calves to the infection during their most resistant phase. If the issue persists, annual vaccination of the calf crop may be required. Cattle susceptible to babesiosis must be vaccinated before entering enzootic areas.

In marginal regions adjacent to enzootic zones, the recommended approach includes pre-outbreak vaccination and post-outbreak chemoprophylaxis. The most effective strategy for controlling babesiosis is to manage and reduce the population of the *Boophilus* tick, the primary vector. In most enzootic areas, the goal is to achieve a balance where tick populations are sufficient to sustain a low-level infection, fostering tolerance to acute babesiosis, and maintaining economically viable disease levels. Rather than aiming for eradication, tick management seeks to achieve this equilibrium.

For one-host ticks that remain on the host for three weeks, dipping once per week is sufficient; however, for multi-host ticks or those with three hosts, dipping twice per week is necessary. Acaricides commonly used include avermectins, carbamates, organophosphates, natural and synthetic pyrethrins, and chlorinated hydrocarbons. Dips and sprays are the primary methods of acaricide application, with dips generally proving more effective. Recent advancements have introduced "pour-ons" and "spot-ons" as alternative application methods. The emergence of tick resistance necessitated the development of these new chemicals. Effective control of vector distribution, particularly in areas of high concentration, requires the identification of affected regions and regulation of livestock movement both into and out of these areas (Estrada-Peña and Salman, 2013).

In babesiosis-endemic areas, chemo-immunization remains the sole method for establishing premunition, as treatments that sterilize the disease leave animals vulnerable to reinfection. Chemo-immunization is also applicable when introducing susceptible cattle into endemic regions, though it must be combined with a robust tick control program to prevent significant losses during severe tick vector challenges. Premunition, a mild, asymptomatic infection caused by a dormant parasite, bolsters the animal's defenses against severe infections by the same Babesia species. Cattle with premunizing parasitemia experience a brief period of sterile immunity following recovery. Subsequent exposure to the parasite, common in endemic areas, results in lifelong immunity. Vaccinated animals exhibit no clinical response to variant strains. Coinfectious immunity or premunition can be induced by inoculating susceptible young calves with live attenuated or virulent organisms, followed by chemotherapy to modify clinical outcomes. In older animals, additional precautions may be necessary when administering vaccinations to avoid complications.

Vaccination against *Babesia bovis* and *Babesia bigemina* has been made available in several countries, typically in the form of monovalent, bivalent, or occasionally trivalent vaccines that may also include *Anaplasma*. These vaccines utilize live organisms, which are rendered avirulent through repeated rapid syringe passages in splenectomized calves. While animals can be vaccinated at any age, the recommended window is between three and nine months. This timing ensures that the vaccine, which provides protection after eight weeks, typically offers lifelong immunity.

Imidocarb has proven to be an effective chemoprophylactic, preventing clinical infection for up to two months while allowing mild subclinical infections as drug levels decline. This approach fosters premunition and immunity. To minimize losses, it is crucial to treat sick cattle promptly and maintain accurate records of treated animals. Delays in treatment can result in failure to recover. Additionally, applying an acaricide to remove ticks from all animals is essential to prevent secondary outbreaks.

Ongoing surveillance of cattle in surrounding farms, including the collection of blood samples from suspicious cases and administering treatment where feasible, is vital. Vaccination remains the most effective measure to prevent the spread of potential outbreaks. All "at risk" animals within the affected zone should be vaccinated with the tick fever vaccine, except those treated with imidocarb or showing symptoms of tick fever.

## 10. Concluding Remark

Bovine babesiosis presents a substantial challenge to livestock health, particularly in areas where tick vectors are prevalent. The disease's complexity, manifesting in both acute and chronic forms, underscores the need for comprehensive management strategies. The economic impact, coupled with the difficulties in controlling the tick populations that transmit the disease, necessitates a multifaceted approach that includes vaccination, vigilant surveillance, and timely treatment. A deep understanding of the pathogenesis of both *Babesia bovis* and *Babesia bigemina* infections is essential for developing targeted interventions to mitigate the severe outcomes associated with these parasites.Effective management and control of bovine babesiosis depend on a nuanced understanding of endemic stability, the complexities of the immune response, and advancements in diagnostic and treatment modalities. The dynamic interplay between host, pathogen, vector, and environment underpins endemic stability, with early exposure in calves playing a crucial role in maintaining this equilibrium. As diagnostic tools and therapeutic strategies continue to evolve, the focus remains on preserving this delicate balance, ensuring that cattle populations in endemic regions can thrive with minimal disease impact. Progress in vaccination, alongside the judicious use of acaricides and chemoprophylaxis, has provided a robust framework for controlling babesiosis. However, the ongoing challenge lies in managing the disease within the context of evolving environmental and genetic factors. Ultimately, the goal is to safeguard livestock health, protect economic livelihoods, and support sustainable agricultural practices through an informed and integrated approach to babesiosis management.

## References

Abdel Hamid, O.M., Radwan, M.E.I. and Abdel Fatah, A., 2014. Biochemical changes associated with babesiosis infested cattle. IOSR J Appl Chem, 7, pp.87-92.

Agrawal, V., Das, G., Jaiswal, A., Jayraw, A. K., Jatav, G. P., Shakya, M., & Jamara, N. (2023). First report on molecular identification of Babesia bigemina in a nervous signs evident naturally infected Holstein-Friesian cattle from Central India. Indian Journal of Animal Research, 57(3), 377-380.

Agrawal, V., Jayraw, A., Shakya, M., Jatav, G., Jamra, N., Singh, N., & Jain, R. (2020). Transplacental transmission of babesiosis in a six-week-old Holstein Friesian calf. Journal of Entomology and Zoology Studies, 8(5), 04-06.

Ali, K. N., & Marif, H. F. (2023). Babesiosis in cattle. One Health Triad, 3, 114-121.

Aziz, K.A., Khalil, W., Mahmoud, M., Hassan, N., Mabrouk, D.M. and Suarez, C.E., 2014. Molecular characterization of babesiosis infected cattle: Improvement of diagnosis and profiling of the immune response genes expression. Glob Vet, 12, pp.197-206.

Bazmani, A., Abolhooshyar, A., Imani-Baran, A. and Akbari, H., 2018. Semi-nested polymerase chain reaction-based detection of Babesia spp. in small ruminants from Northwest of Iran. Veterinary world, 11(3), p.268.

Brown, W.C., Norimine, J., Goff, W.L., Suarez, C.E. and McElwain, T.F., 2006. Prospects for recombinant vaccines against Babesia bovis and related parasites. Parasite Immunology, 28(7), pp.315-327.

Chaudhry, Z.I., Suleman, M., Younus, M. and Aslim, A., 2010. Molecular detection of Babesia bigemina and Babesia bovis in crossbred carrier cattle through PCR. Pakistan Journal of Zoology, 42(2).

Demessie, Y. and Derso, S., 2015. Tick borne hemoparasitic diseases of ruminants: A review. Advances in Biological Research, 9(4), pp.210-224.

Enbiyale, G., Debalke, D., Aman, E., Eedmimand, B. and Abebe, S., 2018. Review on Bovine Babesiosis. Acta Parasitologica Globalis, 9(1), pp.15-26.

Esmaeilnejad, B., Tavassoli, M., Asri-Rezaei, S., Dalir-Naghadeh, B., Mardani, K., Golabi, M., Arjmand, J., Kazemnia, A. and Jalilzadeh, G., 2015. Determination of prevalence and risk factors of infection with Babesia ovis in small ruminants from West Azerbaijan Province, Iran by polymerase chain reaction. Journal of arthropod-borne diseases, 9(2), p.246.

Estrada-Peña, A., & Salman, M. (2013). Current limitations in the control and spread of ticks that affect livestock: A review. Agriculture, 3(2), 221-235.

Fakhar, M., Hajihasani, A., Maroufi, S., Alizadeh, H., Shirzad, H., Piri, F. and Pagheh, A.S., 2012. An epidemiological survey on bovine and ovine babesiosis in Kurdistan Province, western Iran. Tropical animal health and production, 44, pp.319-322.

Feleke, A., Petros, B., Lemecha, H., Wossene, A., Mulatu, W. and Rege, E.J., 2008. Study on monthly dynamics of ticks and seroprevalence of Anaplasma marginale, Babesia bigemina and Theileria mutans in four indigenous breeds of cattle in Ghibe Valley, Ethiopia. SINET: Ethiopian Journal of Science, 31(1), pp.11-20.

Ghadimipour, R., Noaman, V. and Taghizadeh, M., 2020. Prevalence and risk factors of Babesia bovis and Babesia bigemina infection in cattle in northwestern Iran. Veterinary Clinical Pathology The Quarterly Scientific Journal, 14(54), pp.155-168.

Gray, J., Zintl, A., Hildebrandt, A., Hunfeld, K.P. and Weiss, L., 2010. Zoonotic babesiosis: overview of the disease and novel aspects of pathogen identity. Ticks and tick-borne diseases, 1(1), pp.3-10.

Haghi, M.M., Etemadifar, F., Fakhar, M., Teshnizi, S.H., Soosaraei, M., Shokri, A., Hajihasani, A. and Mashhadi, H., 2017. Status of babesiosis among domestic herbivores in Iran: a systematic review and meta-analysis. Parasitology research, 116, pp.1101-1109.

Hamoda, A.F., Radwan, M., Rashed, R. and Amin, A., 2014. Toxic effect of babesiosis in cattle and chemotherapiotic treatment in Egypt. Am J Infect Dis Microbiol, 2, pp.91-6.

Hamsho, A., Tesfamarym, G., Megersa, G. and Megersa, M., 2015. A cross-sectional study of bovine babesiosis in Teltele District, Borena Zone, Southern Ethiopia. J Veterinar Sci Technol, 6(230), p.2.

Herwaldt, B.L., Cacciò, S., Gherlinzoni, F., Aspöck, H., Slemenda, S.B., Piccaluga, P., Martinelli, G., Edelhofer, R., Hollenstein, U., Poletti, G. and Pampiglione, S., 2003. Molecular characterization of a non–Babesia divergens organism causing zoonotic babesiosis in Europe. Emerging infectious diseases, 9(8), p.943.

Homer, M. J., Aguilar-Delfin, I., Telford III, S. R., Krause, P. J., & Persing, D. H. (2000). Babesiosis. Clinical Microbiology Reviews, 13(3), 451-469.

Homer, M.J., Aguilar-Delfin, I., Telford III, S.R., Krause, P.J. and Persing, D.H., 2000. Babesiosis. Clinical microbiology reviews, 13(3), pp.451-469.

Homer, M. J., Bruinsma, E. S., Lodes, M. J., Moro, M. H., Telford III, S., Krause, P. J., ... & Persing, D. H. (2000). A polymorphic multigene family encoding an immunodominant protein from Babesia microti. Journal of Clinical Microbiology, 38(1), 362-368.

Hoyte, H.M.D., 1961. Initial development of infections with Babesia bigemina.

Hunfeld, K. P., Hildebrandt, A., & Gray, J. S. (2008). Babesiosis: Recent insights into an ancient disease. International Journal for Parasitology, 38(11), 1219-1237.

Ijaz, M., Rehman, A., Ali, M.M., Umair, M., Khalid, S., Mehmood, K. and Hanif, A., 2013. Clinico-epidemiology and therapeutical trials on babesiosis in sheep and goats in Lahore, Pakistan.

Jalovecka, M., Sojka, D., Ascencio, M. and Schnittger, L., 2019. Babesia life cycle–when phylogeny meets biology. Trends in parasitology, 35(5), pp.356-368.

Kalani, H., Fakhar, M. and Pagheh, A., 2012. An overview on present situation babesiosis and theileriosis and their distribution of ticks in Iran. Iranian Journal of Medical Microbiology, 5(4), pp.59-71.

Kasozi, K.I., Matovu, E., Tayebwa, D.S., Natuhwera, J., Mugezi, I. and Mahero, M., 2014. Epidemiology of increasing hemo-parasite burden in Ugandan cattle.

Khan, N.A., 2008. Emerging protozoan pathogens. Taylor & Francis.

Laha, R., Das, M., Goswami, A. and Singh, P., 2012. Aclinical case of Babesiosis in across bred cow of Meghalaya. Indian Journal of Animal Research, 46(3), pp.302-305.

Lew, A. and Jorgensen, W., 2005. Molecular approaches to detect and study the organisms causing bovine tick borne diseases: babesiosis and anaplasmosis. African Journal of Biotechnology, 4(4), pp.292-302.

Mahoney, D. F., Wright, I. G., & Goodger, B. V. (1981). Bovine babesiosis: The immunization of cattle with fractions of erythrocytes infected with Babesia bovis (syn B. argentina). Veterinary Immunology and Immunopathology, 2(2), 145-156.

Mohamed, G. and Ebied, M., 2014. Epidemiological studies on bovine Babesiosis and Theileriosis in Qalubia governorate. BVMJ, 27, pp.36-48.

Montenegro-James, S. (1992). Prevalence and control of babesiosis in the Americas. Memórias do Instituto Oswaldo Cruz, 87, 27-36.

Mosqueda, J., Olvera-Ramírez, A., Aguilar-Tipacamu, G. and J Canto, G., 2012. Current advances in detection and treatment of babesiosis. Current medicinal chemistry, 19(10), pp.1504-1518.

Muhanguzi, D., Matovu, E. and Waiswa, C., 2010. Prevalence and characterization of Theileria and Babesia species in cattle under different husbandry systems in western Uganda. Int. J. Anim. Vet. Adv, 2(2), pp.51-58.

Onoja, I.I., Malachy, P., Mshelia, W.P., Okaiyeto, S.O., Danbirni, S. and Kwanashie, G., 2013. Prevalence of babesiosis in cattle and goats at Zaria Abattoir, Nigeria. Journal of Veterinary Advances, 3(7), pp.211-214

Potgieter, F.T. and Els, H.J., 1977. The fine structure of intra-erythrocytic stages of Babesia bigemina.

Potgieter, F.T. and Els, H.J., 1979. An electron microscopic study of intra-erythrocytic stages of Babesia bovis in the brain capillaries of infected splenectomized calves.

Quinn, P.J., Markey, B.K., Leonard, F.C., Hartigan, P., Fanning, S. and Fitzpatrick, E., 2011. Veterinary microbiology and microbial disease. John Wiley & Sons.

Rahbari, S., Nabian, S., Khaki, Z., Alidadi, N. and Ashrafihelan, J., 2008. Clinical, haematologic and pathologic aspects of experimental ovine babesiosis in Iran. Iranian Journal of Veterinary Research, 9(1), pp.59-64.

Riek, R. F. (1964). The life cycle of Babesia bigemina (Smith and Kilborne, 1893) in the tick vector Boophilus microplus (Canestrini). Australian Journal of Agricultural Research, 15(5), 802-821.

Saad, F., Khan, K., Ali, S. and Akbar, N., 2015. Zoonotic significance and prophylactic measure against babesiosis. International Journal of Current Microbiology and Applied Sciences, 4, pp.938-953.

Sajid, M.S., Siddique, R.M., Khan, S.A., Iqbal, Z. and Khan, M.N., 2014. Prevalence and risk factors of anaplasmosis in cattle and buffalo populations of district Khanewal, Punjab, Pakistan. Global Veterinaria, 12(1), pp.146-153.

Schnittger, L., Rodriguez, A.E., Florin-Christensen, M. and Morrison, D.A., 2012. Babesia: a world emerging. Infection, Genetics and Evolution, 12(8), pp.1788-1809.

Scholtens, R.G., Braff, E.H., Healy, G.R. and Gleason, N., 1969. A case of babesiosis in man in the United States.

Schorn, S., Pfister, K., Reulen, H., Mahling, M. and Silaghi, C., 2011. Occurrence of Babesia spp., Rickettsia spp. and Bartonella spp. in Ixodes ricinus in Bavarian public parks, Germany. Parasites & vectors, 4, pp.1-9.

Shahbazi, A., Aboualsoltani, N., Bazmani, A., Khanmohammadi, M., Aboualsoltani, F. and Fallah, E., 2014. Parasitological and molecular study of Babesia microti in rodents of Sarab district (East Azerbaijan of Iran).

Sharma, A.K., Katoch, R.C., Nagal, K.B., Kishtwaria, R.S. and Sharma, S.K., 2000. Bovine babesiosis in Palam Valley of Himachal Pradesh.

Simuunza, M.C., 2009. Differential diagnosis of tick-borne diseases and population genetic analysis of Babesia bovis and Babesia bigemina (Doctoral dissertation, University of Glasgow).

Sitotaw, T., Regassa, F., Zeru, F. and Kahsay, A.G., 2014. Epidemiological significance of major hemoparasites of ruminants in and around Debre-Zeit, Central Ethiopia. Journal of Parasitology and Vector Biology, 6(2), pp.16-22.

Skotarczak, B., 2008. Babesiosis as a disease of people and dogs. Molecular diagnostics: a review. Veterinarni medicina-praha-, 53(5), p.229.

Tavassoli, M., Tabatabaei, M., Mohammadi, M., Esmaeilnejad, B. and Mohamadpour, H., 2013. PCR-based detection of Babesia spp. infection in collected ticks from cattle in west and north-west of Iran. Journal of arthropod-borne diseases, 7(2), p.132.

Taylor, M.A., Coop, R.L. and Wall, R., 2015. Veterinary parasitology. John Wiley & Sons.

Taylor, S. M., Hunter, A. G., & Andrews, A. H. (2004). Ectoparasites, tick and arthropod-borne diseases. In Bovine medicine: Diseases and husbandry of cattle (pp. 740-777). Ames: Blackwell Publisher.

Uilenberg, G., 1995. International collaborative research: significance of tick-borne hemoparasitic diseases to world animal health. Veterinary parasitology, 57(1-3), pp. 19-41.

Uilenberg, G., 2006. Babesia—a historical overview. Veterinary parasitology, 138(1-2), pp.3-10.

Vahedi Nouri, N. and Noaman, V., 2020. The molecular study of babesia species in the cattles of Mazandaran province. Journal of Animal Biology, 12(3), pp.81-90.

Wadhwa, D.R., Pal, B. and Mandial, R.K., 2008. Epidemiological and clinico-therapeutic study of babesiosis in cattle. The Indian Journal of Veterinary Research, 17(2), pp.22-24.

Wagner, G.G., Holman, P. and Waghela, S., 2002. Babesiosis and heartwater: threats without boundaries. Veterinary Clinics: Food Animal Practice, 18(3), pp.417-430.

Weiss, J. B. (1995). DNA probes and PCR for diagnosis of parasitic infections. Clinical Microbiology Reviews, 8(1), 113-130.

Yin, H., Lu, W. and Luo, J., 1997. Babesiosis in China. Tropical animal health and production, 29, pp.11S-15S.

Zahid, I.A., Latif, M. and Baloch, K.B., 2005. Incidence and treatment of theileriasis and babesiasis. Pakistan Veterinary Journal, 25(3), p.137.

Zangana, I.K. and Naqid, I.A., 2011. Prevalence of piroplasmosis (Theileriosis and Babesiosis) among goats in Duhok Governorate. Al-Anbar J Vet Sci, 4(2), pp.50-7.

Zintl, A., Gray, J. S., Skerrett, H. E., & Mulcahy, G. (2005). Possible mechanisms underlying age-related resistance to bovine babesiosis. Parasite Immunology, 27(4), 115-120.

# 5

# Rickettsial Parasite –Anaplasma

***Supriya Sachan[1], Kale Chandrakant Dinkar[1]***
***Rupam Sachan[1], Amit Singh[2] and Saroj Kumar[3]***

[1]*Department of Veterinary Parasitology, College of Veterinary Science and Animal Husbandry, U.P. Pandit Deen Dayal Upadhyaya Pashuchikitsa Vigyaan Vishwavidyalay Evam Go Anusandhan Sansthan, Mathura Uttar Pradesh*
[2]*Department of Veterinary Parasitology, College of Veterinary Science and Animal Husbandry, Acharya Narendra Deva University of Agriculture & Technology, Kumarganj, Ayodhya, Uttar Pradesh*
[3]*Department of Veterinary Parasitology, Faculty of Veterinary and Animal Sciences, Institute of Agricultural Sciences, Banaras Hindu University Varanasi, Uttar Pradesh*

**Order:** Rickettsiales

**Family:** Anaplasmataceae

**Genus:** *Anaplasma*

| **Species** | **Host** | **Vector** | **Epidemiology** |
|---|---|---|---|
| *A. bovis* (*Eimeria bovis*) | Cattle, rabbit | *Amblyomma, Haemphysalis, Ixodes, Rhipicephalus* (*Boophilus*) | Africa, America, Asia |
| *A. caudatum* | Cattle | Unknown | North America |
| *A. centrale* | Cattle | *Haemaphysalis* | Europe, Africa, America, Asia |
| *A. marginale* | Cattle | *Dermacentor, Rhipicephalus* (*Boophilus*) | Cosmopolitan |
| *A. phagocytophilum* (*E. equi, E. phagocytophila,* and *A. phagocytophila*) | Human, equine, sheep, goat, cattle, dog, cat, rodents | *Ixodes, Dermacentor* | Cosmopolitan |

The reclassification of the order *Rickettsiales* was predicated upon comprehensive genetic analyses of 16S rRNA, *groESL*, and surface protein genes. Consequently, organisms within this order were systematically assigned to one of two families: *Anaplasmataceae* and *Rickettsiaceae*. Within the *Anaplasmataceae* family, phylogenetic analyses consistently delineated four genetically distinct clades: (1) *Anaplasma*, (2) *Ehrlichia*, (3) *Wolbachia*, and (4) *Neorickettsia*. Despite the obligate intracellular nature of rickettsial organisms in both families, those classified under *Rickettsiaceae* proliferate freely within the host cell cytoplasm, whereas members of the *Anaplasmataceae* family are confined exclusively to membrane-bound vacuoles within the cytoplasm of host cells.

The first documented cases of anaplasmosis trace back to the late 19$^{th}$ century in South Africa. However, it wasn't until 1910 that the causative agent of the disease was conclusively identified morphologically as "marginal points" within red blood cells by Max Theiler, later named it *Anaplasma marginale*. A year later, he identified another species, *A. centrale*, which caused a milder form of the disease in cattle. During the 1930s, Sanborn, Stiles, and Moc demonstrated the mechanical transmission of *A. marginale* by horse flies and stable flies. In the late 1980s, the life cycle of *A. marginale* was fully elucidated in ticks belonging to the genus *Dermacentor*.

The genus *Anaplasma* belongs to gram-negative bacterial group which are morphologically small (approximately 0.3 μm) and pleomorphic, residing primarily within the cells of the mononuclear phagocytic system, as well as within erythrocytes and platelets of vertebrate hosts. The disease is clinically observable in cattle, though other ruminants, such as water buffalo, bison, African antelopes, and certain deer species, can also develop persistent infections. Due to their intracellular localization, they can be detected in blood smears or aspirates from organs such as the spleen, liver, and bone marrow. Despite being a bacterium, it holds significant importance in veterinary parasitology due to its deceptive resemblance to protozoa. This is because it behaves as an obligate intracellular organism, replicating within host cells, where they aggregate into micro-colonial structures known as morulae. These bacteria are distinct from conventional Gram-negative bacteria due to the absence of a cell wall, rendering them highly susceptible to mechanical stress. While enveloped, they lack leaflet thickening and are devoid of peptidoglycan layers or lipopolysaccharides (LPS).

*Anaplasma marginale* possesses a compact genome of approximately 1.2 megabase pairs, encompassing two gene superfamilies and exhibiting significant genetic heterogeneity among geographically distinct isolates.

These strains have been identified on the basis of differing morphology, protein sequences, antigenic properties, and tick transmission capabilities (Aubry and Geale, 2011). Major surface proteins (MSPs) are integral to *A. marginale's* interactions with host cells, influencing its infectivity by facilitating immune evasion and ensuring its persistence within the host organism throughout its lifespan. Six MSPs have been identified on *A. marginale* derived from bovine erythrocytes (Palmer et al., 1999) and have been found to be conserved in both tick-derived and cell culture-derived organisms (Kocan and de la Fuente, 2003). Following figure highlights the classification of important MSPs:

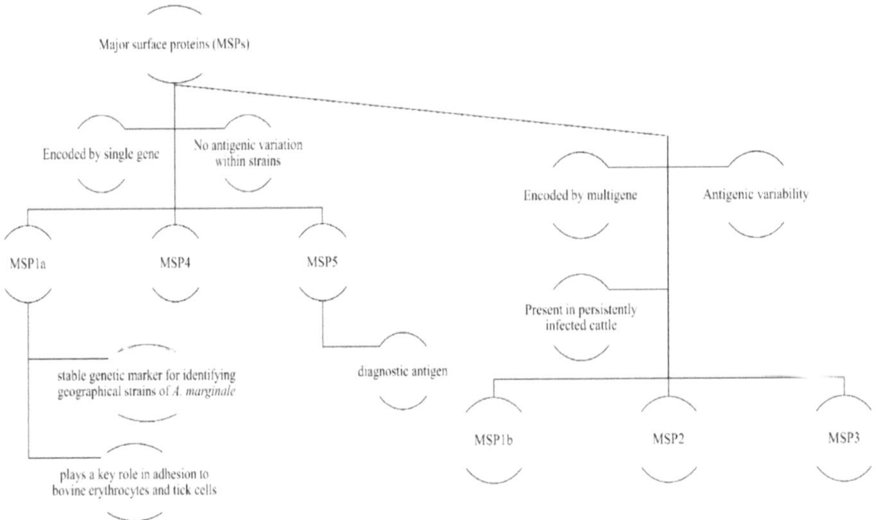


(Salinas-Estrella et al., 2023)

Bovine anaplasmosis is attributed to infection with *Anaplasma marginale*. A closely related yet less virulent organism, *Anaplasma centrale*, is utilized as a live vaccine for cattle in countries such as Israel, South Africa, South America, and Australia (Salinas-Estrella et al., 2023).

## Life-Cycle

Upon infection of erythrocytes by *Anaplasma marginale*, it undergoes intracellular replication, transitioning from a single initial body to form a specialized eight progeny morulae termed as inclusion body. These initial bodies are subsequently released and propagate sequentially within additional erythrocytes, culminating in elevated levels of parasitaemia. Notably, the exit of initial bodies from infected bovine erythrocytes does not induce cellular lysis. The prepatent period varies between 7 to 60 days, during which up to 70% of erythrocytes may become parasitized during acute infection. Instead of undergoing destruction via intravascular lysis, infected erythrocytes are recognized and cleared by macrophages in the spleen, resulting in a reduction of circulating erythrocytes. Following resolution of the acute phase, recovered cattle often remain asymptomatic carriers, serving as reservoirs of infection for susceptible hosts (Kocan et al., 2010).

When ticks feed on infected cattle, they ingest erythrocytes containing initial bodies. Within the tick midgut, the initial bodies are released and proceed to infect the epithelial cells of the intestinal lining, initiating a developmental cycle. One or more cycles of development within the intestinal cells of tick may occur, subsequently leading to the dissemination of *A. marginale* to other tick tissues, including the salivary glands. From these glands, the pathogen is transmitted to vertebrate hosts during tick feeding (Cobaxin-Cárdenas et al., 2019).

The initial morphological manifestation of *A. marginale* within the colony is the reticulate (vegetative) form, which proliferates through binary fission, resulting in large colonies containing hundreds of organisms. The reticulate forms eventually transition into dense forms, which represent the infective stage capable of surviving extracellularly. Cattle become infected with *A. marginale* when the dense form is transmitted via tick salivary secretions during feeding.

## Transmission

The transmission of *Anaplasma* in bovines occurs via both biological and mechanical mechanisms. Biological transmission necessitates the feeding of ticks on carrier hosts, whereas mechanical transmission involves the direct transfer of infected blood without bacterial replication within the vector and contaminated instruments which further complicates control measures. Wild ruminants may act as reservoirs, sustaining the pathogen's circulation within and across herds.

## Biological Transmission

Approximately thirty tick species have been implicated in the dissemination of *Anaplasma*, with *Dermacentor andersoni* and species of *Rhipicephalus microplus* and *Hyalomma marginatum rufipes* being the most extensively studied (Scoles et al., 2008). Transmission of *A. marginale* via *Dermacentor* spp., *R. microplus*, and *R. annulatus* has been well-documented through trans-stadial (across developmental stage) or intra-stadial (within the same stage) pathways (Vimonish et al., 2020).

The interaction between *A. marginale* and its tick vectors is intricate, varying among strains, vector species, and environmental conditions. Trans-stadial and intra-stadial transmission are particularly significant in three-host ticks, as they vacate their host at the conclusion of each developmental stage. Historically, trans-ovarial transmission of *A. marginale* was considered improbable; however, recent findings indicate that larvae of *R. microplus* emerging from infected females are capable of transmitting the pathogen to cattle, despite remaining unfed. This was molecularly confirmed by analysing the variable region of the MSP1a gene (Amaro-Estrada et al., 2020). Critical aspects, such as the influence of temperature and strain variation, warrant further investigation, but these findings underscore the importance of considering transovarial transmission in bovine anaplasmosis control strategies.

Another mode of transmission is transplacental, which may occur during gestation. Carrier cows experiencing immunosuppression often exhibit elevated rickettsemia, facilitating the transplacental passage of *A. marginale* (Zabel and Agusto, 2018). In such cases, some calves exhibit clinical symptoms and may succumb, whereas others remain asymptomatic reservoirs (Rey-Valeirón et al., 2003).

**Mechanical Transmission**

Mechanical transmission involves the transfer of infected blood via contaminated fomites or haematophagous vectors. Although blood-feeding flies play a seemingly minor role in *A. marginale* transmission, they can still facilitate horizontal dissemination of the pathogen in the absence of ticks (Kocan et al., 2010). Haematophagous arthropods, including *Tabanus* spp. (horseflies), *Haematobia irritans* (horn flies), and *Stomoxys calcitrans* (stable flies), have been associated with transmission. However, their efficacy is estimated to be at least 100 times lower than that of tick vectors (Bautista-Garfias et al., 2021).

Within the realm of mechanical transmission, human malpractice plays a significant role, accounting for numerous cases in areas devoid of ticks or where flies are effectively controlled. Routine husbandry practices, such as the reuse of needles during vaccinations, insertion of hormonal implants, and ear-tagging, are common in large herds (Kocan et al., 2010). Empirical evidence has demonstrated that needles used in such procedures are capable of transmitting *Anaplasma* from an infected animal to at least two subsequent hosts (Reinbold et al., 2010).

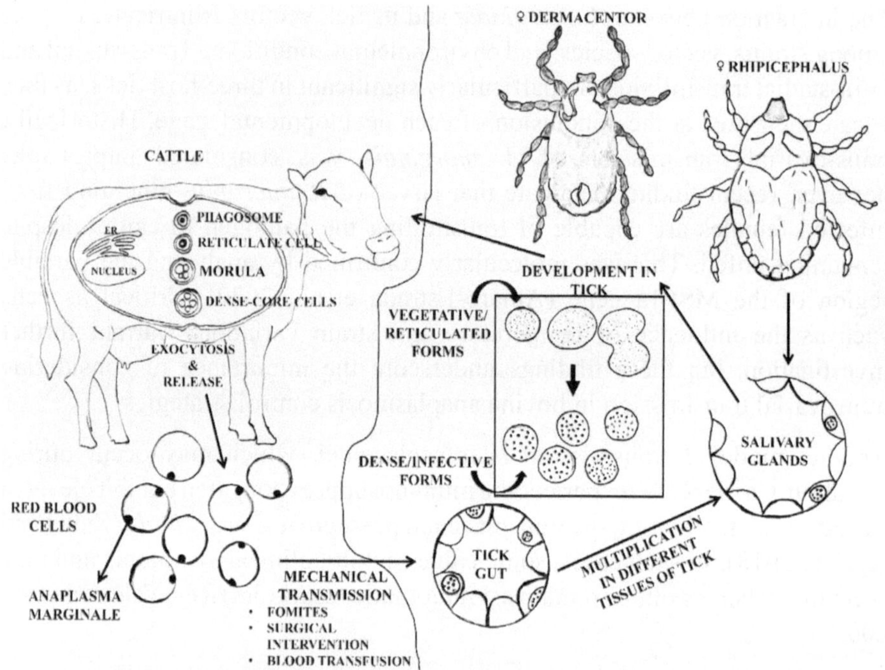


**Fig:** Pictorial representation of both biological and mechanical transmission mechanism in bovine anaplasmosis (Salinas-Estrella et al., 2023)

## Clinical Signs

The common names for an infectious but non-contagious bovine anaplasmosis are:

| | | |
|---|---|---|
| Gall sickness | : | Common name for the disease in South Africa and some other regions |
| Yellow bag | : | Due to icterus yellow discolouration of mucous membranes |
| Yellow fever | : | Due to icterus |
| Tick fever | : | Disease transmitted by ticks |

Anaplasmosis in cattle becomes increasingly severe with age, particularly in animals over two years old. Infections caused by *Anaplasma marginale* are the most severe, with common clinical signs including fever, icterus, anorexia, reduced milk production, and abortion. Anaemia is generally present but varies in severity. In contrast, *Anaplasma centrale* typically causes mild, subclinical infections in cattle, sheep, and goats, though severe anaemia may occur in goats with concurrent diseases. Calves under one year of age usually exhibit mild or asymptomatic infections due to their ability to regenerate red blood cells more rapidly than adults. Older cattle, especially those over two years, are more prone to acute, potentially fatal disease.

Acute anaplasmosis is characterized by fever, lethargy, anorexia, swollen preparotid lymph nodes and progressive anaemia due to the destruction of infected erythrocytes. This results in pale mucous membranes, tachycardia, and dyspnoea as the animal compensates for reduced oxygen delivery. Icterus arises from haemolysis and elevated bilirubin levels, while affected animals may also experience weight loss, weakness, and reduced productivity.

Advanced stages can lead to hypoxia, sudden collapse, and death if untreated. Chronically infected animals may appear clinically normal but act as carriers of the disease, serving as reservoirs for transmission. These carriers are typically asymptomatic but can experience reduced productivity and become sources of infection for susceptible herds.

Anaemia and thrombocytopenia are hallmark clinical features of anaplasmosis, observed across various animal species. *Anaplasma phagocytophilum* typically induces a mild disease in cattle and sheep, with negligible mortality. However, infected pregnant cattle often experience significant reproductive losses due to abortion. Laboratory findings include thrombocytopenia, leukopenia, anaemia, and hyperproteinaemia, with hypoalbuminaemia reported occasionally.

## Epidemiology & Its Contributing Factors

Bovine anaplasmosis is widespread in tropical and subtropical regions, including South and Central America, the United States, southern Europe, Africa, Asia, and Australia. The disease is most prevalent in exotic and crossbred cattle in these regions, driven by the density and distribution of tick vectors and reservoir hosts. Climate change is influencing the geographic distribution of *A. marginale*, with shifts in vector populations extending its range into temperate areas. (Abdisa, 2019)

Age significantly influences the clinical outcome of bovine anaplasmosis. Calves under one year of age exhibit resilience to severe disease, likely due to their rapid erythrocyte regeneration capabilities rather than colostral immunity. Older cattle, particularly those over two years old, are highly susceptible to severe, acute, and sometimes fatal infections. *Bos taurus* breeds are more vulnerable to severe disease than *Bos indicus*. In endemic areas, early exposure during calfhood minimizes losses as animals develop partial immunity.

However, new adult cattle introduced into endemic regions face severe consequences. Chronically infected animals may act as asymptomatic carriers, serving as reservoirs of infection. These carriers can relapse under immunosuppressive conditions, such as corticosteroid treatment, concurrent infections, or splenectomy, contributing to ongoing transmission within herds.

The presence of *A. marginale* is closely associated with environmental conditions conducive to tick survival and reproduction. Global warming is expanding the distribution of vector species, facilitating the pathogen's spread to new regions.

Factors contributing to the prolonged circulation of *Anaplasma* species include the introduction of infected animals into disease-free herds, improper handling of contaminated instruments, and the role of wild ruminants as reservoir hosts. Adult cattle relocated from non-endemic to endemic areas are at higher risk of severe disease and mortality, while calves in endemic regions typically show minimal clinical signs due to early exposure and acquired resistance.

**Bovine Immune Response**

When *Anaplasma marginale* enters a bovine bloodstream through a vector bite, it attaches to RBCs using proteins on its surface, binding to yet-unidentified receptors on the RBC surface. *Anaplasma* form inclusion bodies that release infectious particles, which infect other red blood cells without destroying them. Infected erythrocytes are recognized by macrophages in reticular tissues and vascular sinusoids present in the red pulp of the spleen. Macrophages capture infected red blood cells most effectively at moderate levels of infection but become less efficient when the number of infected cells is very high (Salinas-Estrella et al., 2022). Non-specific phagocytosis has been demonstrated in the spleen and may explain splenomegaly in the infections (Salinas-Estrella et al., 2023).

When the erythrocyte is phagocytized, it initiates antigen processing by denaturing and partially digesting pathogen proteins into short peptides that are presented on MHC class II molecules on the macrophage surface to CD4+ T-helper (Th) cells (Brown et al., 1998). Th cells involved in the immune response include Th1 cells, specialized in the production of interleukin (IL) 2 and interferon gamma, which stimulate the synthesis of IgM and IgG2 synthesis by B cells and activate macrophages (Silvestre et al., 2018). This promotes the production of nitric oxide to kill the parasite.

However, there is also a response of Th2 cells that secrete IL4, IL6 and IL10. The cytokines also stimulate B cells towards the production of IgG1 (Kocan et al., 2010). B cells can also be activated by recognizing an immunogen in its free, untransformed form through their antigen receptors or surface antibodies (Zhao et al., 2016).

Studies indicate that IgG2 is related to the resolution of bovine anaplasmosis, since these antibodies from immune animals are able to opsonize infected erythrocytes and be more rapidly phagocytized (Cantor et al., 1993), unlike IgG1 which is not able to mediate phagocytosis by neutrophils or monocytes (Brown et al., 1998). Interestingly, young cattle under 12 months of age rarely develop severe disease, even when infected, but adult cattle are more vulnerable. Cattle that recover from acute infection remain infected with low rickettsemia, but do not show severe clinical signs of the disease, so they are considered protected against a homologous challenge (Rodríguez-Camarillo et al., 2008), except when there is a concomitant disease inducing a state of immunosuppression. The persistence of the parasite occurs despite the development of a protective immune response.

## Diagnosis

### 1. Conventional Microscopy

The detection of parasite can be done through Giemsa-stained blood smears as a reliable diagnostic method during the acute phase of the disease in clinically infected animals. However, this approach is not suitable for identifying pre-symptomatic or carrier animals.

### 2. Serological Diagnosis

- Complement fixation (CF) test
- Capillary agglutination assay
- Card agglutination test (CAT)
- Indirect fluorescent antibody (IFA) test
- Enzyme-linked immunosorbent assays (ELISAs), such as competitive ELISA (cELISA), indirect ELISA, and dot ELISA

Among these, cELISA and CAT are the most commonly used methods, as recommended by the OIE (2008). However, there is suboptimal sensitivity of serological assays during early infection.

## Competitive Enzyme-Linked Immunosorbent Assay (cELISA)

It is based on monoclonal antibodies targeting the *Anaplasma* MSP5 protein, is currently the most accurate serological assay for identifying *Anaplasma*-infected cattle. While it demonstrates up to 95.6% sensitivity and 98.2% specificity, it cannot differentiate between *A. marginale* and other *Anaplasma* species due to the conserved nature of MSP5. However, there is a chance of low sensitivity during early infections since antibody detection is unreliable during the initial 10 days of infection and only reaches 100% sensitivity from day 13 onward (Aubry and Geale, 2011).

Another limitation is due to the conserved msp5 protein, the test may produce false-positive results in cases of co-infection or exposure to other *Anaplasma* species.

**Card Agglutination Test (CAT)**

This test offers rapid results (within 30 minutes) and is suitable for field or laboratory use (Aubry and Geale, 2011). However, it is limited by non-specific reactions, subjectivity in interpretation, and variability due to differences in antigen preparation.

**Complement Fixation (CF) Test**

While historically used extensively, this test exhibits variable sensitivity (20–60%), poor reproducibility, and a high likelihood of failing to detect carrier or early-stage infections. Its use is no longer recommended due to the risk of false negatives (Aubry and Geale, 2011).

**Indirect Enzyme-Linked Immunosorbent Assay (iELISA)**

An iELISA utilizing a normal red blood cell antigen (negative antigen) and an *Anaplasma marginale*-infected red blood cell antigen (positive antigen) has been demonstrated to reliably detect *A. marginale*-positive sera. The sensitivity was 87.3% and specificity was 98.4% while the cross reactivity was reported with *Anaplasma phagocytophilum*, *Babesia bovis*, and *Babesia bigemina* (Strik et al., 2007).

**Dot Enzyme-Linked Immunosorbent Assay (Dot ELISA)**

The dot ELISA has been proposed as a simpler, faster, and more cost-effective alternative to the iELISA. It is a rapid, inexpensive, and straightforward test to perform with no cross-reactions observed with *Babesia bovis* or *B. bigemina* (Aubry and Geale, 2011).

**Indirect Fluorescent Antibody (IFA) Test**

Although the IFA test has been extensively utilized, its limitations include a low throughput and challenges with nonspecific fluorescence. The test is labour-intensive and only limited number of samples are processed daily. Non-specific fluorescence due to antibodies binding to infected erythrocytes can complicate interpretation (OIE, 2008).

**3. Gold Standard Diagnostic Approach**

The gold standard for determining *A. marginale*-free blood involves sub-inoculation of suspected blood samples into splenectomized calves, which are highly susceptible to the infection. If the donor animal is infected, *A. marginale* can typically be observed in blood smears from the splenectomized calf within 4–8 weeks. However, this method is costly, raises ethical concerns due to the severe illness induced in splenectomized calves, and is no longer widely used for assay validation (Aubry and Geale, 2011).

**4. Lateral Flow Assay (LFA)**

A lateral flow assay for detecting bovine antibodies to *A. marginale* was recently developed using recombinant MSP5 as the antigen and colloidal gold-conjugated monoclonal antibodies for detection. It is a rapid and suitable test for screening cattle from endemic areas. The sensitivity was comparable to cELISA (94–95.5%) while the specificity ranged from 98–98.0% under field conditions. It may occasionally provide false-positive results, particularly in non-endemic areas. Recommended for screening cattle being moved from endemic to disease-free zones (Nielsen et al., 2009).

**5. Molecular Diagnosis**

Nucleic-acid-based diagnostic tests, particularly polymerase chain reaction (PCR), provide high sensitivity in detecting low-level infections in both carrier cattle and tick vectors. PCR assays targeting *A. marginale*-specific DNA sequences have proven valuable in detecting carrier infections. These methods are increasingly employed to validate serological tests and improve diagnostic accuracy. However, some carriers may still be misdiagnosed as negative. The detection efficiency of the test is reported as 24 infected erythrocytes per microliter of blood (equivalent to 0.0001% parasitemia) for conventional PCR, while nested PCR (nPCR) can detect 30 infected erythrocytes per milliliter of blood (corresponding to 0.0000001% parasitemia) (Aubry and Geale, 2011).

Gene of interests for the detection of anaplasmosis are usually MSP4 or MSP1a that have been utilized. Whereas, while targeting MSP5 a cross-reactivity with other *Anaplasma* species is observed (*A. centrale*, *A. ovis*, *A. phagocytophilum*) due to conserved epitopes (Alleman et al., 2006).

**Real-Time PCR (RT-PCR)**

RT-PCR enables sensitive and specific detection and quantification of *A. marginale* DNA. The detection limit observed may be 101 DNA copies or 30 infected erythrocytes per milliliter of blood (Carelli et al., 2007). No cross-reactions is observed with other ruminant haemoparasites, including *A. centrale*, *A. bovis*, and *Theileria buffeli*.

## Control Methods

### a) Vector control and prevention of iatrogenic transmission

Managing vectors both on and off the host is a cumbersome process as it requires significant manual effort and financial resources. Additionally, environmental contamination is an increasing concern, and frequent use of acaricides or insecticides can lead to resistant tick and fly populations respectively. Moreover, it poses the risk of making cattle more vulnerable to infections in endemic regions. Among vector control, tick control is economically more challenging due to the high costs associated with the frequent application of acaricides for effective protection.

An alternative to reduce tick exposure is confining cattle indoors to limit their access to tick-infested pastures. However, this approach is not feasible across all cattle production sectors. In the dairy industry, the use of acaricides is further constrained by licensing limitations and the mandatory waiting period for milk to ensure residue breakdown, making these products practical only for heifers until they reach calving age.

For effective management of fly population sanitation within shed involves regularly cleaning, managing manure, and storing feed properly. Biological control uses natural fly predators like beetles, mites, and parasitoids, which thrive if insecticides are used cautiously. Space sprays and bait are preferable, while residual sprays should be avoided. Releasing parasitoids in early spring or summer can boost their population for effective fly control.

While effective integrated management practices may reduce vector-borne transmission, the risk of iatrogenic transmission remains. Vector control strategies include managing flies, which serve as mechanical vectors, and strictly avoiding the reuse of needles and syringes on multiple animals during herd management. When castration or dehorning is performed surgically, thorough sanitization and disinfection of all instruments between different animals should be a standard practice. Equipment such as tattoo tools, ear tag applicators, nose tongs, prolapse and implant needles should also undergo standard disinfection process among herd. This strict adherence to hygienic practices helps minimizing the risk of fomite-mediated transmission.

In regions where both ticks and biting flies contribute to the transmission of *A. marginale*, it is essential to use products that target both vectors or a combination of treatments. However, vector control alone cannot completely prevent *A. marginale* transmission if blood-contaminated instruments facilitate iatrogenic spread (Kocan et al., 2003).

### b) Premunition

Premunition, a historical control measure, involved vaccinating cattle with whole blood from chronic carriers of bovine anaplasmosis agents. The diluted blood withdrawn from an infected carrier animal can be administered in calves between 6 and 9 months of age. Animals immunized through this method typically develop a mild subclinical condition, offering long-term protection as long as the infection persists. For optimal effectiveness, the procedure should ideally be performed using local strains. While this method requires veterinary supervision and treatment of any clinical symptoms, it poses significant risks. These include potential transmission of other infectious agents and logistical challenges in large-scale application. Due to these concerns and its failure to meet modern safety standards, particularly given the use of biological material, premunition is no longer recommended in many regions, such as the United States.

It is vital to recognize that animals that have undergone successful chemo sterilization which means administering antimicrobial drugs to eliminate *Anaplasma* from carrier animals, preventing further transmission are still completely vulnerable to reinfection with *A. marginale* (Reinbold et al., 2010). As a result, in addition to administering the required antimicrobial treatment at the correct dosage and for the prescribed duration, it is imperative to prevent any exposure to *A. marginale* to maintain the animal's freedom from infection.

### c) Anaplasmosis Free Herds

To sustain a herd free of anaplasmosis all animals—including any new additions—must undergo testing. Any animal that tests positive should be removed from the herd to prevent the spread of infection. Alternatively, some infected cattle may be treated by administering antimicrobial drugs to eliminate *A. marginale* from carrier animals, preventing further transmission. However, this approach can be costly and is currently limited by the lack of approved drugs for this purpose in some regions. Most of the diagnostic tests may occasionally yield false-negative results, sourcing new livestock from low-risk herds which reduces the risk of unintentional introduction of *A. marginale*. The risk of introducing an undetected infected animal into a negative herd can be reduced by incorporating, a two-stage testing approach where in tests are conducted approximately three weeks apart before herd entry. This approach is effective as long as there is no risk of new infections between tests, particularly during periods when vectors are inactive (Aubry and Geale, 2011).

**d) Chemoprophylaxis:** Different chemotherapeutic agents used are mentioned in the table beneath (Maharana et al., 2016; Aubry and Geale, 2011):

| Drug | Approval Status | Usage | Effectiveness | Limitations |
|---|---|---|---|---|
| **Oxytetracycline (OTC)** @ 6-10 mg/kg | Approved in the USA (FDA) | At least 4 days in beef and non-lactating dairy cattle | Reduces parasitemia and clinical signs but does not eliminate persistent infection | Requires regular injections, can be expensive, potential for resistance, withdrawal periods for meat/milk |
| **Chlortetracycline (CTC)** | Approved in the USA (FDA) | Continuous use in medicated feed for controlling active infections in beef cattle | Effective for active infection control but does not clear chronic infections | Requires continuous feeding, risk of resistance |
| **Imidocarb dipropionate** @ 1.5 mg/kg | Used in some regions, but not widespread | In acute anaplasmosis | Limited effect on acute anaplasmosis | Inconsistent efficacy for *A. marginale* |
| **Arsenicals, Antimalarials, Antimony Derivatives, Dyes** | Not widely used | Various chemotherapeutic agents tried | Little to no effect on acute infection | Limited effectiveness and widespread use, rarely employed |
| **Long-acting OTC** @ single dose of 20 mg/kg or two injections @ 20 mg/kg in chronic infection | Not FDA- to eliminate only from carrier animals | Subcutaneous or parenteral injections, multiple doses | Some studies show failure to clear persistent infection | Ineffective in eliminating carrier state, expensive, potential for resistance |
| **High-dose CTC** @ 11 mg/kg | | Administered orally for extended periods (4–6 months) | Some success (79–90%) in clearing persistent infection in steers | Limited success in pregnant cows, higher drug costs, field applicability not proven |
| **Oral CTC** @ 4.4 mg/kg/day | | Administered top-dressed on feed for 45–80 days | Some success in eliminate only from carrier animals, but results vary | Limited clearance in cows, lower plasma levels in pregnant cows, field trials needed |

| Drug | Approval Status | Usage | Effectiveness | Limitations |
|---|---|---|---|---|
| **CTC + Long-acting OTC** | | Combined use of oral CTC with long-acting OTC injections | Some success, but variable results | Need for further field trials, not suitable for all herds |
| **Enrofloxacin** @12.5 mg/kg | Not approved | Two doses subcutaneously, 48 hours apart | In *in-vivo* trial: Inhibit *A. marginale* in a dose-dependent manner in erythrocyte cultures<br>In *in-vitro* trial: Poor efficacy for treating severe experimental *A. marginale* infections and clearing persistent infections in splenectomised calves | Did not eliminate severe infections |

e) **Immunophrophylaxis:** The decision to vaccinate cattle largely depends on the regional epizootiology of bovine anaplasmosis. In areas free of these diseases, vaccination is generally unnecessary unless the cattle originate from endemic regions. In regions with enzootic instability, vaccination is recommended for all calves born outside the tick season. Conversely, in areas with enzootic stability, vaccination is advised only for animals newly introduced from disease-free regions or areas with enzootic instability. Additionally, in such stable regions, vaccination should be performed only in conjunction with an intensive tick control program.

1. Vaccination experiments in older cattle showed that animals with a strong Th1 response (higher IgG2 and more CD4+ T cells than CD8+ T cells) were better protected, while those with weaker Th1 responses often showed severe symptoms. The precise reasons why CD4+ T cells dominate in this immune response are still unclear, but their role is crucial. Current vaccine research focuses on identifying bacterial proteins that activate CD4+ T cells to induce a protective immune response. Combining vaccination with other control measures could provide reliable protection against anaplasmosis in cattle (Salinas-Estrella et al., 2022).

## Live Vaccines

Since the early 20th century live heterologous vaccines against Anaplasma marginale have been utilized to quote Theiler first identified Anaplasma centrale as a distinct organism in South Africa, which was less virulent and could be used to immunize naïve cattle against the more virulent *A. marginale* strain. *A. centrale* continues to be produced as a live vaccine—often as a trivalent combination with *Babesia bovis*, *B. bigemina*, and *A. centrale*—in countries such as South Africa, Australia, Argentina, Brazil, Uruguay, Israel and various parts of South America to protect against *A. marginale*. These vaccines are widely distributed, offering a cost-effective solution for cattle production. In Brazil, two types of attenuated vaccines as mentioned below are commercially available: chilled and frozen (Kessler et al., 2002).

FROZEN VACCINES

ERITROVAC N2® and EMBRAVAC® - HEMOPAR
Preserved in liquid nitrogen, enabling their transportation.
Estimated protection level of approximately 97%
(Kessler et al., 1998)

A second dose may be administered 60 days after the initial vaccination.
Pics ae shorter shelf life, lasting only up to 7 days.
It is recommended to perform serological testing beforehand and only vaccinate individuals who remain seronegative (Kessler et al., 2002).

CHILLED VACCINES
ERITROVAC

shorter shelf life, lasting only up to 7 days.

However, there have been reports of *A. centrale* causing outbreaks with fatal outcomes or failing to provide full immunity against *A. marginale* challenges. Potgieter (1979) stated that while *A. centrale* vaccination attenuates the clinical severity of *A. marginale* infection, it does not prevent infection entirely. Hence, the use of live vaccines should be approached with caution.

Using live virulent *A. marginale* as an immunogen typically involves the sub-inoculation of blood from infected carriers into susceptible animals, coupled with premunition (treatment to prevent acute or fatal anaplasmosis). This method, however, carries uncertainty since the quantity of infected erythrocytes in the inoculum is unpredictable, leading to variable monitoring periods and inconsistent results. Franklin (1967) claimed that in some cases, just 10 µl of infected blood can induce infection with delayed symptoms, while other animals show no clinical signs at all.

Some virulent strains of *A. marginale* have been attenuated through passage in non-natural hosts, such as splenectomized sheep and deer. These attenuated strains have been tested with partial success in several countries, including Mexico, Peru, and Colombia. However, the efficacy of the attenuated strains differs: while the sheep-attenuated strain offers protection similar to that of the live virulent strain, the deer-attenuated strain fails to induce solid immunity. Notably, calves immunized with virulent strains tend to exhibit less severe clinical signs after subsequent artificial or natural challenges compared to those previously immunized with the sheep-attenuated strain. This difference in clinical presentation is thought to result from either a lack of cross-protection between strains or from variations in the antibody responses elicited by the immunizing versus the challenge strains (Salinas-Estrella et al., 2022).

Strains of *A. marginale* with naturally low virulence have also been tested as potential vaccines. Early attempts used the Florida strain, and subsequent trials with local strains have been reported in Australia, Mexico, and Brazil. These efforts generally involve inoculating fresh or frozen infected erythrocytes to induce a mild clinical syndrome (premunition). However, using infected blood presents the risk of transmitting other blood-borne pathogens, such as *Babesia*, *Ehrlichia*, or viruses. For instance, in Australia, bovine leukemia virus (BLV) was inadvertently transmitted to BLV-free cattle, resulting in severe consequences (Silvestre et al., 2016).

2. A key area of progress in bovine anaplasmosis research is the in vitro cultivation of *A. marginale*. Recent studies have shown some success in cultivating *A. marginale* in tick cell lines. This approach has allowed the expression of major surface proteins typical of the erythrocytic stages

of *A. marginale* and *A. centrale*. Although cattle immunized with in vitro-cultured *A. marginale* exhibited an antibody immune response, the protection level achieved was not as robust as expected. The level of protection was comparable to immunization with crude antigens derived from initial bodies against a homologous challenge. Despite these challenges, tick cell lines remain valuable for isolating *A. marginale* from field outbreaks or carriers, providing essential material for further characterization and research (Salinas-Estrella et al., 2022).

## Killed Vaccines

Early attempts at vaccine development, constrained by the inability to utilize *Anaplasma centrale*, employed lyophilized blood containing a high concentration of infected erythrocytes. These were reconstituted with an oil adjuvant and administered to susceptible hosts. However, these early inactivated vaccines proved impractical due to the high erythrocyte stroma content, which was likely linked to cases of neonatal iso-erythrolysis in calves born to vaccinated dams (Rodríguez-Vivas et al., 2017).

Subsequent efforts explored the use of purified initial bodies extracted from bovine erythrocytes. In one study, detergent-solubilized initial bodies combined with Quil-A saponin as an adjuvant were used to immunize adult cattle. Following vaccination, the animals were challenged with a heterologous strain containing 1 × $10^9$ infected erythrocytes. Despite the immunization, the vaccine failed to confer protection (Cobaxin-Cárdenas et al., 2019).

To broaden the antigenic coverage, a vaccine trial conducted in Mexico utilized three strains sharing the major surface proteins MSP1a and MSP4. In this trial, only animals challenged with a combination containing the homologous strain exhibited resistance to infection. All other groups required chemotherapy to prevent mortality under controlled stall conditions (Rodríguez et al., 2000). In contrast, another study using a similar vaccine formulation—identical in adjuvant, antigen composition, and administration route—was conducted under ranch conditions. In this setting, yearling cattle developed specific antibodies as measured by iELISA, against all three strains and were protected against naturally tick-transmitted anaplasmosis for up to a year following a two-dose vaccination protocol (Salinas-Estrella et al., 2022). Although these findings appear contradictory, the discrepancy likely stems from differences in the challenge conditions. The first study employed a high-dose inoculum of $10^8$ freshly reactivated infected erythrocytes under stall conditions, while the second involved gradual natural infection via tick infestation in a ranch environment.

One of the inactivated vaccines for bovine anaplasmosis was produced by University Products LLC, based in Louisiana, USA. According to the manufacturer, while this vaccine did not prevent infection with virulent *A. marginale*, it induced sufficient immunity to protect cattle from the clinical manifestations of the disease. This vaccine was widely used in thousands of animals over the past two decades. These vaccines are no longer available because it failed to protect vaccinated animals against heterologous strains.

3. In the United States, two vaccines are currently available for anaplasmosis. Anaplaz®, the first vaccine developed for cattle by Fort Dodge, was followed by Plazvax®, introduced by Mallinckrodt (later Schering-Plough). Both vaccines function similarly and require two doses, given 4-6 weeks apart, with yearly boosters recommended. These are inactivated vaccines designed to prevent fatalities due to anaplasmosis, although they do not provide complete immunity against the disease. In rare instances, calves born to vaccinated mothers may experience anaemia and death, highlighting the importance of early parasite detection in such cases.

## Next-Generation Vaccines: DNA and Recombinant Proteins

The published *A. marginale* genome has yielded several promising immunodominant and subdominant proteins as vaccine candidates, including outer membrane proteins (OMPs), major surface proteins (MSPs), and proteins associated with the type IV secretion system (TFSS). Early investigations focused on recombinant proteins such as Msp1a, Msp1b, Msp2, Msp3, Msp4, and Msp5 (Salinas-Estrella et al., 2022), assessing their potential for immunization in calves. One of the earliest recombinant DNA vaccine attempts involved coupling the MSP1a gene with promoters from diverse origins into a vaccinia virus vector. When administered to mice, the immunogen elicited a limited production of specific antibodies (McGuire et al., 1984). Another DNA vaccine was engineered by fusing a sequence encoding B- and T-cell epitopes from the MSP1a gene with a BVP22 domain and an MHC class II-targeting motif (foetal liver tyrosine kinase) to enhance antigen presentation by dendritic cells. When administered to 6-month-old calves, this vaccine stimulated proliferative responses, expansion of gamma interferon-positive CD4+ T cells, and IgG responses against the B-cell epitope. However, no live-agent challenge was reported.

In a similar study, recombinant plasmids pET102-MSP1a, pET101-MSP1b, and pRSET-MSP5 were utilized to immunize mice. While the combination of plasmids primarily induced a Th2-type immune response, individual inoculation with pET102-MSP1a triggered a slightly higher IgG response compared to controls (Mwangi et al., 2007).

Recombinant proteins emerged as a viable alternative to DNA vaccines. A blend of rMSP1a, rMSP1b, rMSP4, and rMSP5 proteins formulated with ISCOM and ISCOMATRIX adjuvants successfully induced IgG1 and IgG2 responses in mice. Similarly, recombinant TFSS proteins such as VirB9-1, VirB9-2, and VirB10, linked to MHC class II DRB3 antigens, stimulated antibody production and CD4+ T cell activation in A. marginale-membrane-immunized cattle (Morse et al., 2012). Among these, recombinant VirB9-1 and VirB10, expressed in *Pichia pastoris* and formulated with self-adjuvanting silica vesicles (SV-100), generated significantly higher antibody responses than comparable Quil-A saponin formulations. Furthermore, this preparation elicited robust T-cell responses in calves previously immunized with *A. marginale* outer membranes (Morse et al., 2012).

Various studies have employed diverse immunization strategies, from vector DNA vaccines to recombinant proteins with different adjuvants, testing MSPs, TFSS proteins, and other subdominant antigens in mice, rabbits, or calves. Notably, a mixture of VirB9.1, VirB9.2, VirB10, VirB11, and EfTu proteins induced the desired Th1-type immune response in steers; however, this response did not correlate with protection (Salinas-Estrella et al., 2022).

In addition to conventional targets, subdominant proteins with putative roles in *A. marginale* have been expressed in bacterial systems and evaluated as immunogens. For example, recombinant AM854 (OmpA equivalent) and AM936 (Asp14 equivalent), when formulated with saponin, triggered antigen-specific IgG1 and IgG2 responses in steers. However, vaccinated animals experienced higher levels of rickettsemia and greater packed cell volume losses compared to those immunized with *A. marginale* membrane fragments or negative controls after a tick-borne challenge. In this case, *E. coli*-expressed recombinant antigens led to severe bacteraemia and clinical symptoms, whereas membrane fractions containing native proteins elicited a more favourable Th1-type immune response (Felsheim et al., 2010).

4. The immunization strategy using an eight-branched multiple antigenic peptide (R10K-MAP) derived from MSP1a tandem repeat sequences involved a prime-boost regimen, with the first dose administered subcutaneously, followed by an ear implant containing the antigen and either DEAE-dextran, Quil-A (saponin), or both as adjuvants. Despite inducing antigenicity, the study revealed limited protection in experimental groups, with only one animal per group exhibiting disease resistance (Ducken et al., 2015).

## Genetically Modified Organisms

The transformation of A. marginale was recently achieved using transposon mutagenesis on the *A. marginale* Virginia strain. This mutant exhibit significantly reduced expression of outer membrane protein (Omp) genes, including Omp9, Omp8, Omp7, and Omp6. While this mutant strain can still be transmitted by ticks, its infectivity is markedly diminished in both intact and splenectomized cattle. However, its potential to confer protection against the wild-type Virginia strain or a heterologous challenge was not evaluated (Crosby et al., 2014).

Another vaccine candidate was developed using the St. Maries strain, which underwent transposon-mediated insertion of a 4.5-kb construct containing antibiotic resistance genes for selection and Turbo GFP as a marker. This genetically modified strain, referred to as AmStM-GFP, demonstrates slower growth in culture compared to its parental strain. Immunization with AmStM-GFP resulted in immunity comparable to that induced by *A. centrale*, but it showed some favourable clinical differences. Specifically, vaccinated animals experienced a lower maximum percentage of infected erythrocytes, a smaller decline in packed cell volume, and a longer duration to reach peak bacteremia compared to infections caused by the wild-type AmStM strain (Crosby et al., 2015).

However, the use of live agents presents inherent risks, including the potential transmission of other microorganisms, such as Mycoplasma or viruses, which may contaminate culture systems.

## Acknowledgement

The authors are thankful to 4th Professional, undergraduate Veterinary scholar, Ishan Garg for drawing illustrative figures in this book chapter.

## References

Abdisa, T., 2019. Epidemiology of bovine anaplasmosis. SOJ Vet Sci, 5(1), pp.1-6.

Alleman, A.R., Barbet, A.F., Sorenson, H.L., Strik, N.I., Wamsley, H.L., Wong, S.J., Chandrashaker, R., Gaschen, F.P., Luckschander, N. and Bjöersdorff, A., 2006. Cloning and expression of the gene encoding the major surface protein 5 (MSP5) of Anaplasma phagocytophilum and potential application for serodiagnosis. Veterinary clinical pathology, 35(4), pp.418-425.

Amaro Estrada, I., García-Ortiz, M.A., Preciado de la Torre, J.F., Rojas-Ramírez, E.E., Hernández-Ortiz, R., Alpírez-Mendoza, F. and Rodríguez Camarillo, S.D., 2020. Transmission of Anaplasma marginale by unfed Rhipicephalus microplus tick larvae under experimental conditions. Revista mexicana de ciencias pecuarias, 11(1), pp.116-131.

Aubry, P. and Geale, D.W., 2011. A review of bovine anaplasmosis. Transboundary and emerging diseases, 58(1), pp.1-30.

Bautista-Garfias, C.R., Aguilar-Marcelino, L. and Nogueda-Torres, B., 2023. Myiasis infections in animals and men. Unique Scientific Publishers, 3, pp.20-27.

Brown, W.C., Zhu, D., Shkap, V., McGuire, T.C., Blouin, E.F., Kocan, K.M. et al., 1998. The repertoire of Anaplasma marginale antigens recognized by CD4(+) T-lymphocyte clones from protectively immunized cattle is diverse and includes major surface protein 2 (MSP-2) and MSP-3. Infection and Immunity, 66(11), pp.5414–5422. doi: 10.1128/IAI.66.11.5414-5422.1998.

Camarillo, S.D.R., Ortiz, M.Á.G., Ramírez, E.E.R., Alarcon, G.J.C., De La Torre, J.F.P., Cruz, R.R., Aragón, J.A.R. and Torres, R.A., 2008. Anaplasma marginale Yucatan (Mexico) strain: assessment of low virulence and potential use as a live vaccine. Annals of the New York Academy of Sciences, 1149(1), pp.98-102.

Cantor, G.H., Pontzer, C.H. and Palmer, G.H., 1993. Opsonization of Anaplasma marginale mediated by bovine antibody against surface protein MSP-1. Veterinary immunology and immunopathology, 37(3-4), pp.343-350.

Carelli, G., Decaro, N., Lorusso, A., Elia, G., Lorusso, E., Mari, V., Ceci, L. and Buonavoglia, C., 2007. Detection and quantification of Anaplasma marginale DNA in blood samples of cattle by real-time PCR. Veterinary microbiology, 124(1-2), pp.107-114.

Chapter, O.I.E., 2008. 2.4. 1: bovine anaplasmosis. Manual of standards for diagnostic tests and vaccines for terrestrial animals. Paris: OIE.

Cobaxin-Cardenas, M.E., Díaz, H.A., Avelino, P.O., Salinas-Estrella, E., Preciado-de la Torre, J.F., Quiroz-Castañeda, R.E., Amaro-Estrada, I., Cossío-Bayúgar, R. and Rodríguez-Camarillo, S., 2019. Primer abordaje para la propagación de Anaplasma marginale (MEX-31-096) en células de garrapata Rm-sus. Revista del Centro de Investigación de la Universidad la Salle, 13(51), pp.67-80.

Crosby, F.L., Brayton, K.A., Magunda, F., Munderloh, U.G., Kelley, K.L. and Barbet, A.F., 2015. Reduced Infectivity in cattle for an outer membrane protein mutant of Anaplasma marginale. Applied and environmental microbiology, 81(6), pp.2206-2214.

Crosby, F.L., Wamsley, H.L., Pate, M.G., Lundgren, A.M., Noh, S.M., Munderloh, U.G. and Barbet, A.F., 2014. Knockout of an outer membrane protein operon of Anaplasma marginale by transposon mutagenesis. BMC genomics, 15, pp.1-15.

Ducken, D.R., Brown, W.C., Alperin, D.C., Brayton, K.A., Reif, K.E., Turse, J.E., Palmer, G.H. and Noh, S.M., 2015. Subdominant outer membrane antigens in Anaplasma marginale: conservation, antigenicity, and protective capacity using recombinant protein. PLoS One, 10(6), p.e0129309.

Felsheim, R.F., Chávez, A.S.O., Palmer, G.H., Crosby, L., Barbet, A.F., Kurtti, T.J. and Munderloh, U.G., 2010. Transformation of Anaplasma marginale. Veterinary parasitology, 167(2-4), pp.167-174.

Franklin, T.E. and Huff, J.W., 1967. A proposed method of premunizing cattle with minimum inocula of Anaplasma marginale. Research in Veterinary Science, 8(4), pp.415-418.

Kessler, R.H., Soares, C.O., Madruga, C.R. and Araújo, F.R., 2002. Tristeza parasitária dos bovinos: quando vacinar é preciso. Campo Grande: Embrapa Gado de Corte.

Kocan, K.M., de la Fuente, J., Blouin, E.F., Coetzee, J.F. and Ewing, S.A., 2010. The natural history of Anaplasma marginale. Veterinary parasitology, 167(2-4), pp.95-107.

Kocan, K.M., de la Fuente, J., Guglielmone, A.A. and Meléndez, R.D., 2003. Antigens and alternatives for control of Anaplasma marginale infection in cattle. Clinical microbiology reviews, 16(4), pp.698-712.

Kocan, K.M., de la Fuente, J., Guglielmone, A.A. and Meléndez, R.D., 2003. Antigens and alternatives for control of Anaplasma marginale infection in cattle. Clinical microbiology reviews, 16(4), pp.698-712.

Maharana, B.R., Tewari, A.K., Saravanan, B.C. and Sudhakar, N.R., 2016. Important hemoprotozoan diseases of livestock: Challenges in current diagnostics and therapeutics: An update. Veterinary world, 9(5), p.487.

Morse, K., Norimine, J., Palmer, G.H., Sutten, E.L., Baszler, T.V. and Brown, W.C., 2012. Association and evidence for linked recognition of type IV secretion system proteins VirB9-1, VirB9-2, and VirB10 in Anaplasma marginale. Infection and immunity, 80(1), pp.215-227.

Mwangi, W., Brown, W.C., Splitter, G.A., Davies, C.J., Howard, C.J., Hope, J.C., Aida, Y., Zhuang, Y., Hunter, B.J. and Palmer, G.H., 2007. DNA vaccine construct incorporating intercellular trafficking and intracellular targeting motifs effectively primes and induces memory B-and T-cell responses in outbred animals. Clinical and Vaccine Immunology, 14(3), pp.304-311.

Nielsen, K., Yu, W.L., Kelly, L., Williams, J., Dajer, A., Gutierrez, E., Cruz, G.R., Renteria, T., Bermudez, R. and Algire, J., 2009. Validation and field assessment of a rapid lateral flow assay for detection of bovine antibody to Anaplasma marginale. Journal of Immunoassay and Immunochemistry®, 30(3), pp.313-321.

Palmer, G.H., Rurangirwa, F.R., Kocan, K.M. and Brown, W.C., 1999. Molecular basis for vaccine development against the ehrlichial pathogen Anaplasma marginale. Parasitology today, 15(7), pp.281-286.

Potgieter, F.T., 1979. Epizootiology and control of anaplasmosis in South Africa. Journal of the South African Veterinary Association, 50(4), pp.367-372.

Reinbold, J.B., Coetzee, J.F., Hollis, L.C., Nickell, J.S., Riegel, C.M., Christopher, J.A. and Ganta, R.R., 2010. Comparison of iatrogenic transmission of Anaplasma marginale in Holstein steers via needle and needle-free injection techniques. American journal of veterinary research, 71(10), pp.1178-1188.

Rey-Valeirón CA and Coronado A, 2003. Prevalencia de Anaplasma marginale y anticuerpos específicos en becerros neonatos. Acta Científica Venezolana, 121-126.

Rodríguez, S.D., Ortiz, G. and MA, H.S., 2000. G., Santos Cerda, NA, Aboytes Torre, R. & Cantó Alarcón, GJ: Anaplasma marginale inactivated vaccine: dose titration against a homologous challenge. Comp Immunol Microbiol Infect Dis, 23, pp.239-252.

Rodríguez-Vivas, R.I., Grisi, L., Pérez de León, A.A., Villela, H.S., Torres-Acosta, J.F.D.J., Fragoso Sánchez, H., Romero Salas, D., Rosario Cruz, R., Saldierna, F. and García Carrasco, D., 2017. Potential economic impact assessment for cattle parasites in Mexico. Review. Revista mexicana de ciencias pecuarias, 8(1), pp.61-74.

Salinas-Estrella, E., Amaro-Estrada, I., Cobaxin-Cárdenas, M.E. and Rodríguez-Camarillo, S.D., 2023. Bovine Anaplasmosis: Diagnosis, Treatment and Control Strategies. One Health Triad, Unique Scientific Publishers, Faisalabad, Pakistan, 2, pp.94-101.

Salinas-Estrella, E., Amaro-Estrada, I., Cobaxin-Cárdenas, M.E., Preciado de la Torre, J.F. and Rodríguez, S.D., 2022. Bovine Anaplasmosis: Will there ever be an almighty effective vaccine?. Frontiers in Veterinary Science, 9, p.946545.

Scoles, G.A., Miller, J.A. and Foil, L.D., 2008. Comparison of the efficiency of biological transmission of Anaplasma marginale (Rickettsiales: Anaplasmataceae) by Dermacentor andersoni Stiles (Acari: Ixodidae) with mechanical transmission by the horse fly, Tabanus fuscicostatus Hine (Diptera: Muscidae). Journal of Medical Entomology, 45(1), pp.109–114.

Silvestre, B.T., Silveira, J.A.G., Meneses, R.M., Facury-Filho, E.J., Carvalho, A.U. and Ribeiro, M.F.B., 2016. Identification of a vertically transmitted strain from Anaplasma marginale (UFMG3): molecular and phylogenetic characterization, and evaluation of virulence. Ticks and Tick-borne Diseases, 7, pp.80–84. doi: 10.1016/j.ttbdis.2015.09.001.

Strik, N.I., Alleman, A.R., Barbet, A.F., Sorenson, H.L., Wamsley, H.L., Gaschen, F.P., Luckschander, N., Wong, S., Chu, F., Foley, J.E. and Bjoersdorff, A., 2007. Characterization of Anaplasma phagocytophilum major surface protein 5 and the extent of its cross-reactivity with A. marginale. Clinical and vaccine immunology, 14(3), pp.262-268.

Vimonish, R., Johnson, W.C., Mousel, M.R., Brayton, K.A., Scoles, G.A., Noh, S.M. and Ueti, M.W., 2020. Quantitative analysis of Anaplasma marginale acquisition and transmission by Dermacentor andersoni fed in vitro. Scientific reports, 10(1), p.470.

Zabel, T.A. and Agusto, F.B., 2018. Transmission dynamics of bovine anaplasmosis in a cattle herd. Interdisciplinary perspectives on infectious diseases, 2018(1), p.4373981.

Zhao, L., Mahony, D., Cavallaro, A.S., Zhang, B., Zhang, J., Deringer, J.R. et al., 2016. Immunogenicity of outer membrane proteins VirB9–1 and VirB9–2, a novel nanovaccine against Anaplasma marginale. PLoS ONE, 11, e0154295. doi: 10.1371/journal.pone.0154295.

# 6

# Current Trends in Diagnosis of Haemoprotozoan Infection In Dairy Animals

***Saroj Kumar[1], Kruti Debnath Mandal[2] and Supriya Sachan[3]***

*[1]Department of Veterinary Parasitology, Faculty of Veterinary and Animal Sciences, Institute of Agricultural Sciences, Banaras Hindu University Varanasi, U.P., India*
*[2]Teaching Veterinary Clinical Complex, Faculty of Veterinary and Animal Sciences, Institute of Agricultural Sciences, Banaras Hindu University Varanasi, U.P, India*
*[3]Department of Veterinary Parasitology, College of Veterinary Science and Animal Husbandry, U.P. Pandit Deen, Dayal Upadhyaya Pashuchikitsa Vigyaan Vishwavidyalay Evam Go, Anusandhan Sansthan, Mathura U.P., India*

---

Haemoprotozoan parasites are responsible for causing severe infections in humans as well as animals across the world. The important hemoprotozoan diseases of livestock are trypanosomosis, theileriosis, babesiosis, and anaplasmosis, which are caused by several species of *Trypanosoma*, *Theileria*, *Babesia*, and *Anaplasma*, respectively, in several species of livestock. These diseases caused huge impact on health and productivity of livestock as well as human beings and causes great economic losses to the livestock production in terms of morbidity and mortality worldwide. In India, the annual economic loss has been esteemed in the livestock due to theileriosis, babesiosis and trypanosomosis of Rs 8426 crore, Rs 4000 crore and Rs 4474 core, respectively. The major clinical signs of the haemoprotozoan disease varies from fever, anorexia, anaemia, abortion, and even death in the acute form of infections. The symptomatological treatment is a quite common practice in the field condition to treat the animals suspected with haemoprotozon infection leading to the development of resistance in animals to currently available drugs against haemoprotozoans. The accurate and prompt diagnosis of haemoprotozoan infection is a key to control these diseases. Routine diagnosis of haemoprotozoan infection has been rely on clinical findings and microscopical demonstration of the infective parasitic stages in the blood or tissue fluid smear. Conventional diagnostic techniques such as Microscopical examination techniques and Immunological assay provide the definite clues about parasitic infections in general, but these tests have some limitations. Microscopic examination techniques based on the presence of parasitic stages in the samples, microscopical techniques are highly specific with relatively low sensitivity while Immunological assay such as Complement fixation test (CFT), Card agglutination trypanosomosis test (CATT), Indirect fluorescent antibody test (IFAT) and Enzyme linked immunosorbent assay (ELISA), Immunochromatographic test (ICT) are based mainly on Antigen-Antibody reaction in the blood serum and body fluid and provide information about serodiagnosis of parasitic infections. The main challenge in standardizing these immunological assays is the exiguity of specific non-cross-reactive test reagents. The sensitivity and specificity of these immunological assays for detecting infection specific antibody are not known because very limited comparative evaluations have been available in public domain. Certain parasitic infections may be detected through cell cultures method, however diagnosing the infection by isolating the organisms in the cell culture is a laborious, time-consuming process and frequently fails when using specimens from non-sterile sources. Therefore, the cell culture method is not recommended as a routine laboratory technique for diagnosing most of the haemoparasites, although animal inoculation test is unethical, it is nonetheless a reliable diagnostic method for blood-borne parasites like trypanosomes. In light of these, molecular based diagnostic technique is now the preferred technique for identifying parasites. Most commonly used molecular techniques are Polymerase chain reaction (PCR), Nested PCR, Real-time PCR, Loop-mediated isothermal amplification (LAMP), etc. The ability of nucleic acid-based PCR to detect parasites in blood, tissue or vectors such as ticks with high levels of sensitivity and specificity even in very mild, early and latent phase of infection when the level of parasitaemia is often below the detection limit of commonly used parasitological methods as well as in the evaluation of the efficacy of the particular chemotherapeutic intervention, besides its use in epidemiological study. Further, these techniques can also be used to identify subspecies of parasites. However, recombinant antigens-based ELISAs may be used for routine serodiagnosis of parasitic infections in the field. The molecular-based approaches provide more sensitivity and specificity than the microscopy and serology-based approaches, which greatly increase the probability of specific detection in test samples. The molecular techniques exhibit significant use when dealing with a large number of samples at a much higher sensitivity and they also possess the necessary flexibility for automation and upgradation. However, recent developments in the advancement of new diagnostic tools have opened new opportunities for a significant improvement in parasite detection. Firstly, a number of newer serology-based assays that are highly specific and sensitive have emerged, such as the LAT, IFAT, Immunoblot, Immunochromatographic test (ICT), ELISA, Dot-ELISA, FAST-ELISA etc. using native or recombinant proteins. Secondly, molecular-based approaches such as PCR, real-time PCR, LAMP etc. have shown high potential for use in diagnosis with increased specificity and sensitivity. Thirdly, proteomic technology has also been introduced for the discovery of suitable biomarkers using tissues or biological fluids from the infected host. These techniques can be utilized for early and accurate diagnosis of parasitic diseases as well as to carried out the prevalence studies and make the strategies for control and prevention of diseases of veterinary and zoonotic importance.

## Trypanosomosis

Trypanosomosis is a most important haemo protozoan parasites, caused by a flagellated protozoan parasite *Trypanosoma evansi,* which infects a wide range of domestic animals (camels, horses, donkeys, mules, cattle, buffaloes, dogs, sheep and goats etc.) and human beings in the tropical country. The disease is commonly called as Surra and is transmitted mechanically by biting of blood sucking flies including *Tabanus*, *Stomoxys* and *Haematopota.* The prevalence of surra is higher during monsoon and post monsoon seasons because these seasons are most favourable for the development of these flies, resulting in more disease propagation. However, the cases of surra come across throughout the year. Surra is the most widely distributed pathogenic animal trypanosome, affecting livestock in Asia, Africa and Central and South America. It causes significant economic losses to livestock farmers in terms of morbidity, mortality, abortion, infertility, reduced milk yield and indiscriminate use of drugs against trypanosomes. Presently, *Trypanosoma evansi* infection has been emerging in non-endemic areas and infecting new hosts including occasional cases in humans, raising concerns about the zoonotic potential of this infection. Effective surveillance of *Trypanosoma evansi* infections in India is severely limited due to a lack of sensitive diagnostic tests as well as information on their distribution. Although the level of awareness in veterinarians and diagnostic laboratories concerning *T. evansi* is almost adequate, the lack of diagnostic techniques of high sensitivity hinders quick identification. The microscopic diagnosis of trypanosomosis is usually based on the demonstration of the parasites in the microscopic examination of wet blood film, stained thick/thin smears, lymph node biopsies, joint fluid, and cerebrospinal fluid (in case of nervous signs). The microscopy is the only diagnostic tool in addition to animal inoculation with high specificity and easy to use. However, it has low sensitivity ($1x10^5$ parasites/ml of blood), leading to an erroneous assessment of false negative results, which often even leads to the death of the infected animals in the absence of appropriate treatment. The concentration methods such as microhematocrit centrifugation, quantitative buffy coat technique, and mini-anion-exchange centrifugation technique can detect parasitemia as low as 50 parasites/ml of blood. This limits the utility of microscopy in resource-poor settings. The accurate diagnosis of trypanosomosis is extremely important for identifying the suspected animals for treatment as well as to tracking the prevalence of disease. In light of this fact, recently more attention has been focused on the development of more sensitive and specific immunological and nucleic acid-based test and a number of tests have been described for the diagnosis of surra in livestock animals.

Immunological diagnostic assay is useful for diagnosis of trypanosomosis, can detect antibodies and proteins produced by the immune system in response to parasites. The antibody detection methods include agglutination test, gel diffusion test, counter immunoelectrophoresis, complement fixation test (CFT), card agglutination test (CATT), latex agglutination test (LAT), ELISA, dot- ELISA, western blotting, IFAT etc. The complement fixation test is a very old test and was used successfully in the control and eradication of dourine in North America and the diagnosis of surra in buffalo in the Philippines. The RoTat 1.2 antigen-based card agglutination test standardized for the diagnosis of trypanosomosis caused by *T. evansi* has been extensively used for epidemiological studies. This is RoTat 1.2 antigen-based diagnostic test detect antibodies in the serum that indicate a Type A *T. evansi* infection. These tests include the Card Agglutination Test for *T. evansi* (CATT/*T. evansi*), the Latex Agglutination Test for *T. evansi* (LATEX/*T. evansi*), and the Enzyme-Linked Immunosorbent Assay for *T. evansi* (ELISA/*T. evansi*). The variant antigen type (VAT) of a trypanosome is determined by the VSG, which is highly immunogenic and elicits an antibody response in the host for opsonization, agglutination, and trypanolytic activity. The indirect fluorescent antibody test (IFAT) is both specific and sensitive for the detection of trypanosome antibodies in animals and humans. However, a major problem associated with IFAT is the cross-reactivity between different species of *Tryponosoma* and the requirement of the sophisticated fluorescent microscope. On the contrary, ELISA is quite robust, regardless of the host species. It provides the same range of sensitivity and specificity (90-95%) in the various host species investigated. In field conditions, the antibody-based ELISA (Ab-ELISA) is a better and more sensitive tool to diagnose the chronic stage of trypanosomosis by detecting the

IgG immunoglobulin in established infections. The Ab-ELISA was successfully used to study sero-epidemiology of the surra in cattle and equines in India. A monoclonal antibody-based latex agglutination test has been claimed effective in the diagnosis of surra in domesticated animals under field conditions, which have been reported to be simple, rapid, and cost-effective in field conditions. Some antigen-based ELISAs have been introduced for the detection of circulating trypanosomal invariable antigens and evaluated on a relatively large scale. Recently, a commercial LAT (Suratex) for diagnosis of surra has been developed, but requires further evaluation in field conditions. Currently, several researches have been carried out to search the potential diagnostic antigenic target for the preparation of recombinant antigens such as surface glycoprotein (VSG), invariant trypanosome surface proteins (ISG65, ISG75, ISG100), calflagin (CLF) etc. Other possible antigen candidate molecules include various intracellular proteins including trypanosome derived proteases. These molecules are currently under investigation for their diagnostic potential. A variety of nucleic acid-based molecular techniques has been developed to improve the specificity and sensitivity of the detection of parasites. Several DNA based diagnostic assays have been developed which include the use of species-specific primers, PCR, nested PCR, real-time PCR, LAMP and DNA probes. Numerous target regions of parasites have been used to design primers such as kinetoplast, repetitive sequence DNA and ribosomal DNA. The internal transcribed spacer (ITS) region of rRNA has highly conserved sequences that may be specific to each species and is present in 100– 200 copies per genome. Primers have been designed to identify several trypanosome species by conventional PCR. Tandem repeat domain of GM6 (cytoskeletal protein) has diagnostic value and its usefulness as seroepidemiological studies of surra has been evaluated among water buffaloes. PCR based on ISG75 gene can be useful in the detection of the carrier status of surra in animals. With the use of generic primers in semi-nested PCR targeting variable region of 18s rDNA gene followed by the restriction fragment length polymorphism (RFLP) approach, it is possible to differentiate between important trypanosome species infecting bovines with mixed infections. However, requirements for trained manpower and sophisticated equipment have restricted its use for wide application in the endemic areas. The isothermal reactions, such as LAMP have been developed by many workers using primers designed from different target genes for diagnosis of *Trypanosoma* and nucleic acid sequence-based amplification (NASBA), have recently been developed for the diagnosis of trypanosomosis; however, the techniques have increased application only for detection of human cases. More recently, proteome and secretome analysis providing valuable clues for the identification of immunodominant antigens of

*T. evansi* for detection. Aptamers are single stranded nucleic acid probes that can be selected from a large random library. They are analogues to antibodies in their mode of action and can be coupled to biotin or gold particles and used for development of lateral flow assay for detection of trypanosoma infection. The anti-trypanosome VSG-specific aptamers have been developed in recent years and showed affinities in sub nanomolar range, binding to structurally conserved epitopes of VSG. In recent years, research developments are underway in many laboratories to search potential biomarkers using proteomic approach for development of diagnostics for trypanosomosis. Initially, cytokines and chemokines have been targeted for search of effective diagnostic biomarker molecules. The monitoring of level of various cytokines and chemokines (monocyte chemo attractant protein- 1, macrophage inflammatory protein 1-α, CCL-3, CXCL-8, IL-8, and IL-1ß) could prove valuable tools to determine the stage of Trypanosoma infection in affected hosts. To explore potential biomarkers for diagnosis of trypanosomosis, there is a need of considerable further research experimental studies in this area.

## Theileriosis

Theileriosis is haemoprotozoan diseases caused by *Theileria* sp, an obligate intracellular protozoan parasite that infect both wild and domestic Bovidae throughout the world (some species may also infect small ruminants). In India, bovine tropical theileriosis is caused by *Theileria annulata*. It is a lymphoproliferative disease with high mortality and morbidity in cattle. The group of parasites referred as *Theileria sergenti/ T. buffeli/ T. orientalis* cause mild or asymptomatic disease in cattle and well known as bovine benign theileriosis. The infective stages (sporozoite) of diseases are transmitted by ixodid ticks, and have complex life cycles in both vertebrate and invertebrate hosts. Certain *Ixodid* ticks, such as *Hyalomma anatolicum anatolicum, H. m. marginatum,* and *H. a. excavatum* known to transmit *T. annulata,* are found in semi-arid areas while other genera of ticks like *Amblyomma, Rhipicephalus,* and *Haemaphysalis* were acts as vector in the transmission of benign *Theileria* species. The subclinical infection in cattle with *T. annulata* in endemic regions produces chronic carrier state and serves as potent sources of infection for ticks. Therefore, latent infections are important in the epidemiology of theileriosis. The diagnosis of acute case of theileriosis is based on clinical signs, knowledge of disease and vector distribution as well as microscopic examination of Giemsa-stained thin blood and lymph node and tissue impression smears. The *Theileria* spp. infections are diagnosed by the detection of piroplasms in erythrocytes or schizonts in white blood cells. However, microscopic examination needs expertise for detection of piroplasm/

schizonts in subclinical or chronic infections because parasitemia is often extremely low and may be missed. An immunological test such as indirect fluorescent antibody test (IFAT) is widely used to detect antibodies to *Theileria annulata*. Both schizont and piroplasmic antigen can be used in this purpose. Although, IFAT provides good sensitivity and easy to perform but now a days not followed due to reduced specificity. Enzyme-linked immunosorbent assays (ELISA) using recombinant proteins of *T. annulata* merozoite surface 1 antigen (Tams1) and the *T. annulata* macroschizont stage protein (TaSP), a heat-shock 70 antigen for *Theileria*. sp. (China) and *T. uilenbergi* immunodominant protein (TuIP) are being used to detect antibodies in infected animals. These ELISAs provide higher sensitivity (>95%) and specificity as compare to the IFAT. Both tests were commercially available with high sensitivity, but the IFA tests were discontinued due to specificity issues. However, both are still being used in research. A rapid lateral flow device has been developed by using recombinant TaSP antigen of *T. annulata* which did not show any cross reactivity with other heamoparasites of cattle. The most important advantages of ELISAs are used as a high throughput, cheap and fast method to screen and diagnose large numbers of samples. In current time, molecular based assay has been considered as most preferred method for detection of *Theileria* species by targeting specific genes and species-based oligonucleotide primers. Several studies documented that PCR is more sensitive and specific than other conventional diagnostic techniques in determining piroplasm-carrier animals. Different variants of PCR such as conventional PCR, PCR-RFLP, nested-PCR, PCR followed by dot blotting, capillary blotting or slot-blotting and hybridisation using radio-isotope labelled probes. The latter was improved by the non-radioactive reverse line blot method that used chemiluminescence and probe based real-time PCR methods, SYBR green real-time PCR assays, loop-mediated isothermal amplification (LAMP) assays, pan-FRET based and high-resolution melt analysis, can be followed for fast and accurate diagnosis of the infection. Reverse Line Blot (RLB) micro array is a recently developed technique that uses oligonucleotide probe to detect and identify *Theleria* and/ *Babesia* simultaneously that by specifically amplifying the rRNA gene of V4 hypervariable region of all *Babesia* and *Theileria* species. The obtained PCR products are then hybridized to nitrocellulose membrane, onto which different species-specific oligonucleotide probes are covalently linked. This assay has been extensively used in epidemiological surveys in various countries. In all these cases, the presence of parasitic genetic material can be directly confirmed using the molecular assay, implying the existence of live parasites in the animal at the time of sample collection. The developments in the molecular assays from conventional PCR to nested PCR to real time PCR has been led to improvements in sensitivity, quantification and speed up the detection of parasites. Meanwhile, other techniques such as reverse line blot, bead arrays, pan-FRET assays and high-resolution melt analysis offers the possibility of detecting of multiple species or genotypes at the same time.

## Babesiosis

Babesiosis is one of important parasitic diseases caused by an intraerythrocytic protozoans of the genus *Babesia* and it is characterized by haemolytic anemia and fever, with occasional hemoglobinuria and death. Babesiosis affecting the many species of mammals with a major impact on cattle, equine, dogs and man with worldwide distribution. Babesiosis was first reported in 1888 by Viktor Babes in Romania who detected the presence of round, intra-erythrocytic bodies in the blood of infected cattle. Many species of *Babesia* such as *Babesia bovis*, *B. bigemina* and *B. divergens* are affecting the bovine population. In India, *Babesia bigemina* is the important species infecting cattle. Bovine babesiosis is clinically characterized by increased in body temperature, high rate of pulse, and respiration with decreased appetite and disinclination to movement. In acute infection, hemoglobinurea and hemolytic anemia are most important clinical signs and may results in fatal outcome in absence of chemotherapy. Different diagnostic techniques have been implemented to diagnose bovine babesiosis, usually the microscopic detection of *Babesia* parasites has been considered as the gold standard for the diagnosis of acute babesiosis. However, the low sensitivity of the microscopic technique is the major drawback which may give false negative detection of parasites in the chronic case of infection as well as in the carrier animals. In such case, Immunological assays such as the Indirect Fluorescent Antibody Test (IFAT), Enzyme-Linked Immunosorbent Assay (ELISA) and Immunochromatography Test (ICT) have been utilized to detect the babesiosis in animals exposed to *Babesia* or the passive transfer of antibodies by colostrum in their calves. Recently an immunochromatographic test (ICT) has been developed to detect antibodies to *B. bovis* and *B. bigemina* in serum samples from infected cattle, based on *B. bovis* recombinant merozoite surface antigen (rMSA-2c) and the recombinant C-terminal portion of the *B. bigemina* rhoptry-associated protein-1 (rRAP1/CT). The concordance rates to detect the *B. bovis* antibodies by these ICT assays were 92.3% and 90.3% as compared to the ELISA and IFAT assays, respectively; whereas the for *B. bigemina* antibodies for both assays were 96.8% and 92.5%, respectively, and no detection of antibody cross-reactivity was reported. These immune assays often are described as diagnostic tests lacking specificity, are time-consuming and difficult to perform. Furthermore, the major disadvantages of these assays are the cross-reactivity among the species and also in genus level for species-specific diagnosis and unable to discriminate between previous exposure and current infection. Therefore, Nucleic acids-based molecular assays have been developed in recent past years with increased and sensitivity and specificity to detect *B. bovis*, *B. bigemina* and *B. divergens*. Different types of PCR assays have developed for the identification of persistent infection through the direct detection of the parasite genomic DNA. PCR enables to detect the parasitaemia as low as a few organisms per ml of infected blood sample.

Several molecular epidemiological surveys have been conducted throughout the various countries to detect and genetically characterize *Babesia* parasites present in apparently healthy animals. Recently, various PCR and nested PCR assays targeting *B. bovis* rhoptry-associated protein-1 (BbovRAP-1); *B. bovis* spherical body protein 2 (BboSBP2); *B. bovis* spherical body protein 4 (BboSBP4); *B. bovis* Merozoite Surface Antigen (MSA-1); *B. bigemina* Apical Membrane Antigen-1 (BbiAMA-1) and *B. bigemina* rhoptry-associated protein-1a (BbiRAP-1a) have proven to be a powerful tool for epidemiological investigations in apparently healthy, persistently infected cattle in Pakistan, Ghana, Mongolia, Brazil, Egypt, South Africa, Myanmar, Thailand, Syria, India, and the Philippines.

The Real-time PCR is useful, especially in early stage of infection when results of serological tests are negative, and the blood smear does not reveal the pathogen or where the distinction between inter-erythrocytic forms of related organisms, viz., *Theileria* sp. and *Plasmodium* sp. required. The quantitative PCR (qPCR) has developed as a TaqMan probe assay in a duplex format for the diagnosis of *B. bovis* and *B. bigemina*. In addition to this, *B. divergens* was also detected by a fluorescence resonance energy transfer (FRET) probe, which allowed to differentiate among the species of bovine i.e., *B. bovis*, *B. bigemina* and *B. divergens*. Reverse line blot (RLB) is a more sensitive method than PCR since it is able to detect extremely low parasitemia levels and simultaneously identify *Theileria* and *Babesia* species using specific oligonucleotide probes. Another, Loop mediated isothermal amplification (LAMP) assay has developed as a rapid, cheap, highly sensitive and specific assay which utilized for diagnosis of babesiosis infection in animals. Therefore, LAMP assay has considered as a promising molecular diagnosis tool for diagnosis of bovine babesiosis in a field because it is a simple diagnostic method, which does not require sophisticated equipment, and can be used for screening large number of samples. Recent development in molecular biology has improve the possibility of correct and specific diagnosis of hemoprotozoan diseases. The 18S rDNA gene (18s rDNA, SSU rDNA) is one of the frequently used molecular markers in diagnostic and epidemiological studies, PCR assay targeting SSU rRNA of

*B. bigemina* has been used for detection of low-level *B. bigemina* infection in yaks at the yak rearing tracts of Himalayas. However, none of these molecular based assays could be considered better than another. The utilization of these molecular assays in diagnostic varies as per the need of studies.

## Anaplasmosis

Anaplasmosis is a severe tick-borne disease of ruminants caused by *Anaplasma marginale*. *Anaplasma* sp. is an obligate intra-erythrocyte rickettsial organism, distributed worldwide. Bovine anaplasmosis occurs in tropical and subtropical regions mainly due to *A. marginale* and *Anaplasma centrale.* The clinical outbreaks of bovine anaplasmosis are associated with *Anaplasma marginale* infection and disease is characterized by fever, anaemia, jaundice, abortion, and even death of animal in some cases whereas *Anaplasma centrale* is capable of producing a moderate degree of anaemia, but clinical outbreaks in the field are extremely rare. The new species of *Anaplasma, A. phagocytophilum* and *A. bovis* have been reported that can infect the cattle, but do not cause clinical disease. The rodents act as primary reservoir and wild ruminants particularly cervids served as important reservoirs of infection for *A. marginale*, *A. Phagocytophilum, A. bovis* and *A. ovis*. The diagnosis of anaplasmosis is similar to babesiosis, it can be made by microscopic examination of Giemsa stained thick and thin blood smear for detection of *Anaplasma* parasites. This method is suitable for clinically infected animals during the acute phase of the disease, but it is not reliable for detecting infection in pre-symptomatic or carrier animals. In such condition, we have to diagnose the disease by adopting immunological or molecular assay. Several immunological and molecular assays have been established to detect this rickettsia in carrier animals, where parasitemia is low. Among immunological assays, card agglutination test (CAT), enzyme linked immunosorbent assay (ELISA) and competitive ELISA (cELISA) and indirect ELISA (iELISA) have been widely used for anaplasmosis field evaluations. A c-ELISA using a recombinant antigen termed major surface receptor protein 5 (rMSP5) and MSP5-specific monoclonal antibody (MAb) has proven very sensitive and specific for detection of *Anaplasma*-infected animals. However, none of these tests have been developed to identify antibodies in milk and due to the presence of similar B epitopes in anaplasma species, the available immunological assay shows the cross reactivity among the different species. Nowadays, nucleic acid based diagnostic assay such as such as RLB, PCR, PCR-ELISA, nested PCR, and real-time PCR are used for diagnosis of anaplamosis with high levels of sensitivity and specificity.

## Conclusion

Accurate and prompt diagnosis of the parasitic agents is most crucial steps for control of the haemoprotozoan infections. Microscopic examination methods are still the cheapest and gold standard methods for detection of haemoparatozoan parasites, although has low sensitivity and requires expertise. The immunological assays such as CFT, CATT, IFAT, ELISA, ICT etc. become more popular assays for diagnosis of hemoprotozoan diseases because these have higher sensitivity. However, the efficiency of these assays depends on the use recombinant or parasite-derived diagnostic antigen molecules to detect circulating antibodies against the parasites. The major limitations of immunological assays are cross reactivity with the antibodies of different species or among the species of parasites, which have been documented by various workers. Now a days, nucleic acid based molecular assays are developed for detection of parasites, which are very sensitive, specific and reliable. Various types of PCR such as PCR-RAPD, PCR-AFLP, nested PCR, real time PCR, qPCR, LAMP etc. have been developed and utilized to diagnosed, differentiate the species and genotypic characterization as well as for epidemiological studies of haemoprotozoan parasites. Although these techniques are performed by using expensive reagents and sophisticated equipment. Therefore, the future advance research has been focused for develops new technology which are user friendly, performed without the need of expensive apparatus and have high sensitivity and specificity. These advanced techniques help in accurate and prompt diagnosis of parasitic infections, which improves the control and management strategies of these infections and controlling the emergence of drug resistance.

## References

Abdo, J., Kristersson, T., Seitzer, U., Renneker, S., Merza, M., Ahmed, J., (2010). Development and laboratory evaluation of a lateral flow device (LFD) for the serodiagnosis of Theileria annulata infection. Parasitol. Res. 107, 1241–1248.

AbouLaila, M.; Yokoyama, N.; Igarashi, I., (2010). Development and evaluation of a nested PCR based on spherical body protein 2 gene for the diagnosis of Babesia bovis infection. Vet. Parasitol.,169, 45–50.

Alhassan, A., Govind, Y., Tam, N.T., Thekisoe, O.M.M., Yokoyama, N., Inoue, N., et al., (2007). Comparative evaluation of the sensitivity of LAMP, PCR and in vitro culture methods for the diagnosis of equine piroplasmosis. Parasitol. Res. 100, 1165–1168.

Almeria, S., Castella, J., Ferrer, D., Ortuno, A., Estrada Peña, A. and Gutierrez, J.F. (2001) Bovine piroplasms in minorca (Balearic Islands, Spain): A comparison of PCR based and light microscopy detection. Vet. Parasitol., 99: 249-259.

Amerault, T.E., Rose, J.E., Roby, T.O., (1972). Modified card agglutination test for bovine anaplasmosis: evaluation with serum and plasma from experimental and natural cases of anaplasmosis. Proc. 76th Annu. Meet. U.S. Anim. Health Assoc. 1, 736–744

Aubry, P. and Geale, D.W. (2011) A review of bovine anaplasmosis. Transbound. Emerg. Dis., 58(1): 1-30.

Babes, V., Sur l' hémoglobinurie bactérienne du boeuf. . C. R. Acad. Sci., 1888, 107, 692-694.

Bawm, S.; Htun, L.L.; Maw, N.N.; Ngwe, T.; Tosa, Y.; Kon, T.; Kaneko, C.; Nakao, R.; Sakurai, T.; Kato, H.; et al. (2016). Molecular survey of Babesia infections in cattle from different areas of Myanmar. Ticks Tick Borne Dis, 7, 204–207.

Bazarusanga, T., Geysen, D., Vercruysse, J., Marcotty, T., 2008. The sensitivity of PCR and serology in different Theileria parva epidemiological situations in Rwanda. Vet. Parasitol. 154, 21–31.

Behera, S.K., Banerjee, P.S., Garg, R. and Maharana, B.R. (2012) A case of Babesia equi. Indian Vet. J., 89(12): 87-88.

Bhat, S.A.; Singh, H.; Singh, N.K.; Rath, S.S., (2015). Molecular detection of Babesia bigemina infection in apparently healthy cattle of central plain zone of Punjab. J. Parasit. Dis., 39, 649–653.

Bishop, R., Sohanpal, B., Kariuki, D.P., Young, A.S., Nene, V., Baylis, H., et al., (1992). Detection of a carrier state in Theileria parva-infected cattle by the polymerase chain reaction. Parasitology, 104, 215–232.

Bock, R.; Jackson, L.; de Vos, A.; Jorgensen, W. (2004). Babesiosis of cattle. Parasitology, 129 Suppl, S247-269.

Burridge, M.J., (1971). Application of the indirect fluorescent antibody test in experimental East Coast fever (Theileria parva infection in cattle). Res. Vet. Sci.,12, 338–341.

Burridge, M.J., Kimber, C.D., (1972). The indirect fluorescent antibody test for experimental East Coast fever (Theileria parva infection of cattle). Evaluation of a cell culture schizont antigen. Res. Vet. Sci. 13, 451–455.

Buscher, P., Mumba, N.D., Kabore, J., Lejon, V. and Robays, J. (2009). Improved Models of mini anion exchange centrifugation technique (mAECT) and modified single centrifugation (MSC) for sleeping sickness diagnosis and staging. PLoS Negl. Trop. Dis., 3: e471.

Chaisi, M.E., Janssens, M.E., Vermeiren, L., Oosthuizen, M.C., Collins, N.E., Geysen, D., (2013). Evaluation of a real-time PCR test for the detection and discrimination of Theileria species in the African buffalo (Syncerus caffer). PLoS ONE 8, e75827.

Chaudhry, Z.I.; Suleman, M.; Younus, M.; Aslim, A. (2010). Molecular Detection of Babesia bigemina and Babesia bovis in crossbred carrier cattle through PCR. Pakistan J. Zool., 42, 201–204.

Collins, N.E., Allsopp, M.T., Allsopp, B.A., (2002). Molecular diagnosis of theileriosis and heartwater in bovines in Africa. Trans. R. Soc. Trop. Med. Hyg. 96, S217–S224.

Courtney, J.W., Kostelnik, L.M., Zeidner, N.V. and Massung, R.F. (2004). Multiplex Real-Time PCR for detection of Anaplasma phagocytophilum and Borrelia burgdorferi. J. Clin. Microbiol., 42: 3164-3168.

Criado-Fornelio, A.; Buling, A.; Asenzo, G.; Benitez, D.; Florin-Christensen, M.; Gonzalez-Oliva, A.; Henriques, G.; Silva, M.; Alongi, A.; Agnone, A.; et al. (2009). Development of fluorogenic probe-based PCR assays for the detection and quantification of bovine piroplasmids. Vet. Parasitol, 162, 200–206.

Cringoli, G., Otranto, D., Testini, G., Buono, V., Di Giulio, G., Traversa, D., Lia, R., Rinaldi, L., Veneziano, V., Puccini, V., (2002). Epidemiology of bovine tick-borne diseases in Southern Italy. Vet. Res. 33, 421–428.

De Wall, D.T., (2000). Anaplasmosis control and diagnosis in South Africa. Ann. N. Y. Acad. Sci. 916, 474–483.

Deborggraeve, S. and Buscher, P. (2010). Molecular diagnostics for sleeping sickness: What is the benefit for the patient? Lancet Infect. Dis., 10: 433-439.

Desquesnes, M., Dargantes, A., Lai, D.H., Lun, Z.R., Holzmuller, P. and Sathaporn, J. (2013) Trypanosoma evansi and surra: A review and perspectives on transmission, epidemiology and control, impact, and zoonotic aspects. Biomed. Res. Int., 2013: 321237.

Dreher U.M., De La Fuente J., Hofmann-Lehmann R., Meli M.K., Pusteria N., Kocan K.M., Woldehiwet A., Regula G., Staerk K.D.C. (2005). Serologic cross reactivity between Anaplasma marginale and Anaplasma phagocytophilum. Clin. Vaccine. Immunol., 12, 1177–1183.

Duffy, T., Cura, C.I., Ramirez, J.C., Abate, T., Cayo, N.M., Parrado, R., Bello, Z.D., Velazquez, E., Muñoz-Calderon, A., Juiz, N.A., Basile, J., Garcia, L., Riarte, A., Nasser, J.R., Ocampo, S.B., Yadon, Z.E., Torrico, F., de Noya, B.A., Ribeiro, I. and Schijman, A.G. (2013) Analytical performance of a multiplex real-time PCR assay using TaqMan probes for quantification of Trypanosoma cruzi satellite DNA in blood samples. PLoS Negl. Trop. Dis., 7(1): e2000.

Dumler J.S., Barbet A.F., Bekker C.P., Dasch G.A., Palmer G.H., Ray S.C., Rikihisa Y., Rurangirwa F.R. (2001). Reorganization of genera in the Families Rickettsiaceae and Anaplasmataceae in the order Rickettsiales: unification of some species of Ehrlichia with Anaplasma, Cowdria with Ehrlichia, and Ehrlichia with Neorickettsia, descriptions of five new species combinations and designation of Ehrlichia equi and 'HGE agent' as subjective synonyms of Ehrlichia phagocytophila. Int. J. Syst. Evol. Microbiol., 51, 2145–2165.

Durrani, A.Z., Ahmad, M., Ashraf, M., Khan, M.S., Khan, J.A., Kamal, N. and Mumtaz, N. (2008). Prevalence of theileriosis in buffaloes and detection through blood smear examination and polymerase chain reaction test in district Lahore. J. Anim. Plant Sci., 18(2-3): 59.

Figueroa, J.V.; Chieves, L.P.; Johnson, G.S.; Buening, G.M. (1992). Detection of Babesia bigemina-infected carriers by polymerase reaction amplification. J. Clin. Microbiol., 30, 2576–2582.

Gale, K.R., Dimmock, C.M., Gartside, M. and Leatch, G. (1996). Anaplasma marginale: Detection of carrier cattle by PCR-ELISA. Int. J. Parasitol., 26(10): 1103-1109.

Gasser, R.B. (2006). Molecular tools - Advances, opportunities and prospects. Vet. Parasitol., 136(2): 69-89.

Geysen, D., Delespaux, V. and Geerts, S. (2003). PCR-RFLP using Ssu-rDNA amplification as an easy method for species-specific diagnosis of Trypanosoma species in cattle. Vet. Parasitol., 110: 171-180.

Gill, B.S. (1991). Trypanosomes and Trypanosomiases of Indian Livestock.ICAR, NewDelhi. pp. 191.

Guan, G., Moreau, E., Liu, J., Hao, X. and Luo, J. (2010). Molecular evidence of experimental transmission to sheep by Haemaphysalis qinghaiensis and Haemaphysalis longicornis. Parasitol. Int., 59: 265-267.

Gubbels, J.M., de Vos, A.P., van der Weide, M., Viseras, J., Schouls, L.M., de Vries, E. and Jongejan, F. (1999). Simultaneous detection of bovine Theileria and Babesia species by reverse line blot hybridization. J. Clin. Microbiol., 37(6): 1782-1789.

Gubbels, M.J., d'Oliveira, C., Jongejan, F., (2000). Development of an indirect Tams1 enzyme-linked immunosorbent assay for diagnosis of Theileria annulata infection in cattle. Clin. Diagn. Lab. Immunol. 7, 404–411.

Gutierrez, C.; Desquesnes, M.; Touratier, L.; Büscher, P. (2010). Trypanosoma evansi: Recent Outbreaks in Europe. Vet. Parasitol., 174, 26–29.

Hadush Birhanu, H., Roge, S., Simond, S., Baelmans, R., Gebrehiwot, T., Maria Goddeeris, B., Buscher, P., (2015). Surra Sero K-SeT, a new immunochromatographic test for serodiagnosis of Trypanosoma evansi infection in domestic animals. Vet. Parasitol., 211, 153–157.

Heidarpour Bami, M., Haddadzadeh, H.R., Kazemi, B., Khazraiinia, P., Bandehpour, M., Aktas, M., (2009). Molecular identification of ovine Theileria species by a new PCR-RFLP method. Vet. Parasitol. 161, 171–177.

Hofmann-Lehmann R., Meli M.L., Dreher U.M., Gönczi E., Deplazes P., Braun U., Engels M., Schüpbach J., Jörger K., Thoma R., Griot C., Stärkk.D.C., Willi B., Schmidt J., Kocan K.M., Lutz H. (2004). Concurrent infections with vectorborne pathogens associated with fatal haemolytic anemia in a cattle herd in Switzerland. J. Clin. Microbiol., 42, 3775–3780.

Iseki, H.; Alhassan, A.; Ohta, N.; Thekisoe, O.M.; Yokohama, N.; Inoue, N.; Nambota, A.; Yasuda, J.; Igarashi, I., (2007). Development of a multiplex loop-mediated isothermal amplification (mLAMP) method for the simultaneous detection of bovine Babesia parasites. J. Microbiol. Methods, 71, 281–287.

Jeong, W., Kweon, C.H., Kang, S.W., Paik, S.G., (2003). Diagnosis and quantification of Theileria sergenti using TaqMan PCR. Vet. Parasitol. 111, 287–295.

Kiara, H., Jennings, A., Bronsvoort, B.M., Handel, I.G., Mwangi, S.T., Mbole-Kariuki, M., et al., (2014). A longitudinal assessment of the serological response to Theileria parva and other tick-borne parasites from birth to one year in a cohort of indigenous calves in western Kenya. Parasitology 141, 1289–1298.

Kim, C., Iseki, H., Herbas, M.S., Yokoyama, N., Suzuki, H., Xuan, X., Fujisaki, K., Kawazu, S. and Igarashi, I. (2007). Development of TaqMan-based real-time PCR assays for diagnostic detection of Babesia bovis and Babesia bigemina. Am. J. Trop. Med. Hyg., 77(5): 837-841.

Kim, C.M., Blanco, L.B., Alhassan, A., Iseki, H., Yokoyama, N., Xuan, X., et al., (2008a). Diagnostic real-time PCR assay for the quantitative detection of Theileria equi from equine blood samples. Vet. Parasitol. 151, 158–163.

Kim, C.M.; Blanco, L.B.; Alhassan, A.; Iseki, H.; Yokoyama, N.; Xuan, X.; Igarashi, I., (2008b). Development of a rapid immunochromatographic test for simultaneous serodiagnosis of bovine babesiosis caused by Babesia bovis and Babesia bigemina. Am. J. Trop. Med. Hyg., 78, 117–121.

Kim, J., Alvarez Rodriguez, A., Li, Z., Radwanska, M., Magez, S., (2024). Recent Progress in the Detection of Surra, a Neglected Disease Caused by Trypanosoma evansi with a One Health Impact in Large Parts of the Tropic and Sub-Tropic World. Microorganisms. 12, 44. doi.org/10.3390/microorganisms12010044

Knowles, D., Torioni de Echaide, S., Palmer, G.H., McGuire, T.C., Stiller, D., McElwain, T.F., (1996). Antibody against an Anaplasma marginale MSP5 epitope common to tick and erythrocytes stages identifies persistently infected cattle. J. Clin. Microbiol. 34, 2225–2230.

Kohli, S., Atheya, U.K. and Thapliyal, A. (2014). Prevalence of theileriosis in cross-bred cattle: Its detection through blood smear examination and polymerase chain reaction in Dehradun district, Uttarakhand, India, Vet. World, 7(3): 168-171.

Krause, P.J., Telford, S.R. 3rd, Ryan, R., Conrad, P.A., Wilson, M., Thomford, J.W. and Spielman, A. (1994). Diagnosis of babesiosis: Evaluation of a serologic test for the detection of Babesia microti antibody. J. Infect. Dis.,169: 923-926.

Kumar, R., Sethi, K., Batra, K., Kumar, S., Jain, S., and Kumar, S. (2023). Exploring the potential of invariable surface glycoprotein (ISG65) as promising antigen for diagnosis of Trypanosoma evansi infection. Vet. Parasitol., 314, 109866

Kumar, R., Sethi, K., Gaur, D.K., Goyal, S.K., Kumar, S., Jain, S., and Kumar, S. (2022). Use of recombinant calflagin protein as a potential candidate for diagnosis of Trypanosoma evansi infection. Vet. Parasitol., 310, 109776

Kumar, V., Kaur, P., Wadhawan, V.M., Pal, H., Sharma, H. and Kumar, P. (2015). Theileriosis in cattle: prevalence and seasonal incidence in Jalandhar district of Punjab (India). International J. Recent Scientific Res .6: 2998-2999.

Kundu, K., Tewari, A.K., Kurup, S.P., Baidya, S., Rao, J.R. and Joshi, P. (2013). Sero-surveillance for surra in cattle using native surface glycoprotein antigen from Trypanosoma evansi. Vet. Parasitol., 196: 258-264.

Kurup, S.P. and Tewari, A.K. (2012). Induction of protective immune response in mice by a DNA vaccine encoding Trypanosoma evansi beta tubulin gene. Vet. Parasitol., 187: 9-16.

Lanham, S.M. and Godfrey, D.G. (1970). Isolation of salivarian trypanosomes from man and other mammals using DEAE-cellulose. Exp. Parasitol., 28: 521-534.

Liu, A., Guan, G., Du, P., Gou, H., Liu, Z., Liu, J., Ma, M., Yang, J., Li, Y., Niu, Q., Ren, Q., Bai, Q., Yin, H. and Luo, J. (2012). Loop-mediated isothermal amplification (LAMP) method based on two species-specific primer sets for the rapid identification of Chinese Babesia bovis and B. bigemina. Parasitol. Int., 61(4): 658-563.

Liu, A., Guan, G., Du, P., Gou, H., Zhang, J., Liu, Z., et al., (2013). Rapid identification and differentiation of Theileria sergenti and Theileria sinensis using a loop-mediated isothermal amplification (LAMP) assay. Vet. Parasitol. 191, 15–22.

Liu, A., Guan, G., Du, P., Liu, Z., Gou, H., Liu, J., et al., (2012). Loop-mediated isothermal amplification (LAMP) assays for the detection of Theileria annulata infection in China targeting the 18S rRNA and ITS sequences. Exp. Parasitol. 131, 125–129.

Liu, Z., Wang, Z., Yin, H., Luo, J., Zhang, B., Kullmann, B., et al., (2010). Identification of Theileria uilenbergi immunodominant protein for development of an indirect ELISA for diagnosis of ovine theileriosis. Int. J. Parasitol. 40, 591–598.

Luckins, A.G. (1988). Trypanosoma evansi in Asia. Parasitol. Today. 4, 137-142.

Miranda, J., Bakheit, M.A., Liu, Z., Yin, H., Mu, Y., Guo, S., et al., (2006). Development of a recombinant indirect ELISA for the diagnosis of Theileria sp. (China) infection in small ruminants. Parasitol. Res. 98, 561–567.

Mitashi, P., Hasker, E., Lejon, V., Kande, V., Muyembe, J.J., Lutumba, P. and Boelaert, M. (2012). Human African trypanosomiasis diagnosis in first-line health services of endemic countries, a systematic review. PLoS Negl. Trop. Dis., 6(11): e1919.

Mtshali, M.S. and Mtshali, P.S. (2013). Molecular diagnosis and phylogenetic analysis of Babesia bigemina and Babesia bovis hemoparasites from cattle in South Africa. B.M.C. Vet. Res., 9: 154.

Mugasa, C.M., Laurent, T., Schoone, G.J., Kager, P.A., Lubega, G.W. and Schalling, H.D. (2009). Nucleic acid sequence-based amplification with oligochromatography for detection of Trypanosoma brucei in clinical samples. J. Clin. Microbiol., 47: 630-635.

Mugasa, C.M., Schoone, G.J., Ekangu, R.A., Lubega, G.W., Kager, P.A. and Schalling, H.D.F. (2008). Detection of Trypanosoma brucei parasites in blood samples using realtime nucleic acid sequence-based amplification. Diagn. Microbiol. Infect. Dis., 61: 440-445.

Nadeem, A., Aslam, A., Chaudhary, Z.I., Ashraf, K., Saeed, K., Ahmad, N., Ahmed, I. and Rehman, H.U. (2011). Indirect fluorescent antibody technique-based prevalence of surra in equines. Pak. Vet. J., 31(2): 169-170.

Ndao M. (2009). Diagnosis of Parasitic Diseases: Old and New Approaches. Interdisciplinary Perspectives on Infectious Diseases. doi:10.1155/2009/278246

Nguyen, T., Ruttayaporn, N., Goto, Y., Kawazu, S., Sakurai, T., Inoue, N. (2015). A TeGM6-4r antigen-based immunochromatographic test (ICT) for animal trypanosomosis. Parasitol Res., 114:4319–4325.

Nielsen, K., Smith, P., Gall, D., T. de Echaide, S., Wagner, G., Dajer, A., (1996). Development and validation of an indirect enzyme immunoassay for detection of antibody to Anaplasma marginale in bovine sera. Vet. Parasitol. 67, 133–142.

Niu, Q., Luo, J., Guan, G., Ma, M., Liu, Z. and Liu, A. (2009). Detection and differentiation of ovine Theileria and Babesia by reverse line blotting in China. Parasitol. Res., 104: 1417-1423.

Njiru, Z.K., Mikosza, A.S., Matovu, E., Enyaru, J.C., Ouma, J.O., Kibona, S.N., Thompson, R.C. and Ndung'u, J.M. (2008). African trypanosomiasis: Sensitive and rapid detection of the sub-genus Trypanozoon by loop-mediated isothermal amplification (LAMP) of parasite DNA. Int. J. Parasitol., 38: 589-599.

O.I.E. (2010) Bovine babesiosis. In: Terrestrial Manual. Vol. 1. Ch. 2.4. Office International Des Epizooties, World Health Organization for Animal Health, Paris, France. p1-15.

Odongo, D.O., Sunter, J.D., Kiara, H.K., Skilton, R.A., Bishop, R.P., (2010). A nested PCR assay exhibits enhanced sensitivity for detection of Theileria parva infections in bovine blood samples from carrier animals. Parasitol. Res. 106, 357–365.

OIE, 2014. Manual of Diagnostic Tests and Vaccines for Terrestrial Animals, vol. 1–2, seventh ed. Office International Des Epizooties, Paris.

Oura, C.A.L., Bishop, R.P., Wampande, E.M., Lubega, G.W. and Tait, A. (2004). Application of a reverse line blot assay to study the haemoparasites in cattle in Uganda. Int. J. Parasitol., 34(5): 603-613.

Papadpoulos, B., Perie, N.M. and Uilenberg, G. (1996). Piroplasms of domesticated animals in the Macedonia region of Greece. Serological cross reactions. Vet. Parasitol., 63(4): 41-56.

Parthiban, M., Saranya, R., Magesh, M. and Raman, M. (2010). Detection of Theileria parasite in cattle of Tamil Nadu using nested PCR. Tamil Nadu J. Vet. Anim. Sci., 6(4): 162-165.

Perera, P.K., Gasser, R.B., Firestone, S.M., Smith, L., Roeber, F., Jabbar, A., (2014). Semi-quantitative multiplexed-tandem PCR for the detection and differentiation of four Theileria orientalis genotypes in cattle. J. Clin. Microbiol. doi:10.1128/JCM.02536-14.

Pienaar, R., Latif, A.A., Thekisoe, O.M.M., Mans, B.J., (2013). Protein gene candidates for the qualitative molecular detection of Theileria parva in African buffalo (Syncerus caffer) using the real-time SYBR green polymerase chain reaction. Proceedings of the 1st Annual Conference on Advances in Veterinary Science Research, Singapore.

Pienaar, R., Potgieter, F.T., Latif, A.A., Thekisoe, O.M.M., Mans, B.J., (2011a). Mixed Theileria infections in free-ranging buffalo herds: implications for diagnosing Theileria parva infections in Cape buffalo (Syncerus caffer). Parasitology 138, 884–895.

Pienaar, R., Potgieter, F.T., Latif, A.A., Thekisoe, O.M.M., Mans, B.J., (2011b). The HybridII assay: a sensitive and specific real-time hybridization assay for the diagnosis of Theileria parva infection in Cape buffalo (Syncerus caffer) and cattle. Parasitology 138, 1935–1944.

Randall, R. and Schwartz, S.C. (1936). A survey for the incidence of surra in the Philippine islands. Vet. Bull. US Army, 30: 99-108.

Ranjithkumar, M., Saravanan, B.C., Yadav, S.C., Kumar, R., Singh, R. and Dey, S. (2014). Neurological trypanosomiasis in quinapyramine sulfate-treated horses - A breach of the blood-brain barrier? Trop. Anim. Health Prod., 46: 371-377.

Rayulu, V.C., Singh, A. and Chaudhri, S.S. (2007). Monoclonal antibody-based immunoassays for detection of circulating antigens of Trypanosoma evansi in buffaloes. Ital. J. Anim. Sci., 6: 907-910.

Reetha, T.L., Thomas, K.S. and Babu, M. (2012). Occurrence of haemoprotozoan infection in bovines. Int. J. Appl. Biores., 13: 1-2.

Reinbold J.B., Coetzee J.F., Sirigireddy K.R., Ganta R.R. (2010). Detection of Anaplasma marginale and A. phagocytophilum in bovine peripheral blood samples by duplex real-time reverse transcriptase PCR assay. J. Clin. Microbiol., 48, 2424–2432.

Renneker, S., Kullmann, B., Gerber, S., Dobschanski, J., Bakheit, M.A., Geysen, D., et al., (2008). Development of a competitive ELISA for detection of Theileria annulata infection. Trans bound. Emerg. Dis. 55, 249–256.

Ristic, M. In Diseases of Cattle in the Tropics, Firts Edition ed. Ristic, M.; McIntyre, I., Eds.; Martinus Nijhoff Publishers: The Hague, 1981; Vol. 6, pp 443-468.

Ros-García, A., Nicolás, A., García-Pérez, A.L., Juste, R.A. and Hurtado, A. (2012). Development and evaluation of a real-time PCR assay for the quantitative detection of Theileria annulata in cattle. Parasit. Vectors., 5: 171.

Rudramurthy, G.R., Sengupta, P.P., Balamurugan, V., Prabhudas, K. and Rahman, H. (2013). PCR based diagnosis of trypanosomiasis exploring invariant surface glycoprotein (ISG) 75 gene. Vet. Parasitol., 193: 47-58.

Salih, D.A., Ali, A.M., Liu, Z., Bakheit, M.A., Taha, K.M., El Imam, A.H., et al., (2012). Development of a loop-mediated isothermal amplification method for detection of Theileria lestoquardi. Parasitol. Res. 110, 533–538.

Salim, B., Bakheit, M.A., Sugimoto, C., (2013). Rapid detection and identification of Theileria equi and Babesia caballi by high-resolution melting (HRM) analysis. Parasitol. Res. 112, 3883–3886.

Sanmartin, J.G., Nagore, D., Garciaperez, A.L., Juste, R.A. and Hurtaldo, A. (2006). Molecular diagnosis of Theleria and Babesia species infecting cattle in Northern Spain using reverse line blot microarrays. BMC Vet. Res., 2: 16-21.

Saravanan, B.C., Bansal, G.C., Manigandan, L., Sankar, M., Ravindran, R. and Rao, J.R. (2011). Development of a non-radioactive probe generated by RAPD-PCR for the detection of Theileria annulata. Indian J. Anim. Sci., 81(11): 1089-1092.

Saravanan, B.C., Das, S.J., Tewari, A.K., Sankar, M., Kataktalware, M.A. and Ramesha, K.P. (2013). Babesia bigemina infection in yak (Poephagus grunniens L.): Molecular detection and characterization. Vet. Parasitol., 194: 58-64.

Schindler, R., Wokatsch, R., (1965). Versuche zur differenzierung der Theilerien spezies des rindes durch serologische unterschungen. Tropenmed. Parasitol., 16, 85-87.

Schnittger, L., Yin, H., Qi, B., Gubbels, M.J., Beyer, D., Niemann, S., et al., (2004). Simultaneous detection and differentiation of Theileria and Babesia parasites infecting small ruminants by reverse line blotting. Parasitol. Res. 92, 189–196.

Seitzer, U., Bakheit, M.A., Salih, D.E., Ali, A., Haller, D., Yin, H., et al., (2007). From molecule to diagnostic tool: Theileria annulata surface protein TaSP. Parasitol. Res. 101, S217–S223

Shyma, K.P., Gupta, S.K., Singh, A. and Chaudhri, S.S. (2011). Latex agglutination test for detection of trypanosomosis in equines. J. Vet. Parasitol., 25(2): 132-134.

Shyma, K.P., Gupta, S.K., Singh, A. and Chaudhri, S.S. (2012). Efficiency of monoclonal antibody based latex agglutination test in detecting Trypanosoma evansi under field condition for improving the productivity in buffaloes. Buffalo Bull., 31: 163-172.

Sibeko, K.P., Oosthuizen, M.C., Collins, N.E., Geysen, D., Rambritch, N.E., Latif, A.A., et al., (2008). Development and evaluation of a real-time polymerase chain reaction test for the detection of Theileria parva infections in Cape buffalo (Syncerus caffer) and cattle. Vet. Parasitol. 155, 37–48.

Singh, H., Mishra, A.K., Rao, J.R. and Tewari, A.K. (2007a). A PCR assay for detection of Babesia bigemina infection using clotted blood in bovines. J. Appl. Anim. Res., 32: 201-202.

Singh, H., Mishra, A.K., Rao, J.R. and Tewari, A.K. (2007b). Seroprevalence of babesiosis in cattle and buffaloes by indirect fluorescent antibody test. J. Vet. Parasitol., 21(1): 1-4.

Singh, H., Mishra, A.K., Rao, J.R. and Tewari, A.K. (2009). Comparison of indirect fluorescent antibody test (IFAT) and slide enzyme linked immunosorbent assay (SELISA) for diagnosis of Babesia bigemina infection in bovines. Trop. Anim. Health Prod., 41(2): 153-159.

Singh, V. and Tewari, A.K. (2012) Bovine surra in India: An update. Rumin. Sci., 1(1): 1-7.

Sivakumar, T.; Altangerel, K.; Battsetseg, B.; Battur, B.; AbouLaila, M.; Munkhjargal, T.; Yoshinari, T.;Yokoyama, N.; Igarashi, I., (2012). Genetic detection of Babesia bigemina from Mongolian cattle using apical membrane antigen-1 gene-based PCR technique. Vet. Parasitol., 187, 17–22.

Sivakumar, T.; Kothalawala, H.; Abeyratne, A.S.; Vimalakumar, S.C.; Meewawe, A.S.; Hadirampela, D.T.; Puvirajan, T.; Sukumar, S.; Kuleswarakumar, K.; Chandrasiri, A.D.N.; et al. (2012). A PCR-based survey of selected Babesia and Theileria parasites in cattle in Sri Lanka. Vet. Parasitol., 190, 263–267.

Sivakumar, T.; Okubo, K.; Igarashi, I.; de Silva, W.K.; Kothalawala, H.; Silva, S.S.P.; Vimalakumar, S.C.; Meewewa, A.S.; Yokoyama, N., (2013). Genetic diversity of merozoite surface antigens in Babesia bovis detected from Sri Lankan cattle. Infect. Genet. Evol., 19, 134–140.

Sivakumar, T.; Okubo, K.; Takemae, H.; Simking, P.; Jittapalapong, S.; Igarashi, I.; Yokoyama, N. (2016). Genetic diversity and antigenic variation of Babesia bovis merozoite surface antigens (MSA-1) in Thailand. Infect. Genet. Evol., 41, 255–261.

Skilton, R.A., Bishop, R.P., Katende, J.M., Mwaura, S., Morzaria, S.P., (2002). The persistence of Theileria parva infection in cattle immunized using two stocks which differ in their ability to induce a carrier state: analysis using a novel blood spot PCR assay. Parasitology 124, 265-276.

Stik, N.I., Alleman, A.R., Barbet, A.F., Sorenson, H.L., Wansley, H.L., Gaschen, F.P., Luckschander, N., Wong, S., Chu, F., Foley, J.E., Bjoersdorff,A., Stuen, S., Knowles, D.P. (2007). Characterization of Anaplasma phagocytophilum major surface protein 5 and the extent of its cross-reactivity with A. marginale. Clin. Vac. Immunol., 14: 262-268.

Swai, E.S., Karimuribo, E.D., Kambarage, D.M., Moshy, W.E., Mbise, A.N., (2007). A comparison of seroprevalence and risk factors for Theileria parva and T. mutans in smallholder dairy cattle in the Tanga and Iringa regions of Tanzania. Vet. J. 174, 390–396.

Tassi, P., Carelli, G., Ceci, L., (2002). Mediterranean environment: a clinical, serological, and hematological study. Ann. N. Y. Acad. Sci. 969, 314–317.

Teal, A.E., Habura, A., Ennis, J., Keithly, J.S. and MadisonAntenucci, S. (2012). A new real-time PCR assay for improved detection of the parasite Babesia microti. J. Clin. Microbiol., 50(3): 903-908.

Terkawi, M.A., Thekiso, O.M., Katsande, C. and Igarashi, I. (2011). Serological Survey of Babesia bovis and Babesia bigemina in cattle of South Africa. Vet. Parasitol., 182: 337-342. 9. Parida, M., Sannarangaiah, S., Dash, P.K., Rao, P.V. and Morita, K. (2008) Loop mediated isothermal amplification (LAMP): A new generation of innovative gene amplification technique; Perspectives in clinical diagnosis of infectious diseases. Rev. Med. Virol., 18(6): 407-421.

Terkawi, M.A.; Alhasan, H.; Huyen, N.X.; Sabagh, A.; Awier, K.; Cao, S.; Goo, Y.K.; Aboge, G.; Yokoyama, N.; Nishikawa, Y.; et al. (2012). Molecular and serological prevalence of Babesia bovis and Babesia bigemina in cattle from central region of Syria. Vet. Parasitol., 187, 307–311.

Terkawi, M.A.; Huyen, N.X.; Shinuo, C.; Inpankaew, T.; Maklon, K.; Aboulaila, M.; Ueno, A.; Goo, Y.K.; Yokoyama, N.; Jittapalapong, S.; et al. (2011). Molecular and serological prevalence of Babesia bovis and Babesia bigemina in water buffaloes in the northeast region of Thailand. Vet. Parasitol., 178, 201–207.

Tewari, A.K., Mishra, A.K. and Rao, J.R. (2000). Isolation and purification of cationic proteins from microaerophilus stationary phase culture supernatants of Babesia bigemina. J. Appl. Anim. Res., 18: 41-48.

Tewari, A.K., Rao, J.R., Mishra, A.K. and Yadav, M.P. (2005). Recent trends in the diagnosis of trypanosomosis (surra) in domesticated animals. Proc. Natl. Acad. Sci. India, 75(B): 121-133.

Tewari, A.K., Ray, D., Mishra, A.K. and Bansal, G.C. (2001). Identification of immunodominant polypeptides common between Babesia bigemina and Theileria annulata. Indian J. Anim. Sci., 71: 679-680.

Thekisoe, O.M., Rambritch, N.E., Nakao, R., Bazie, R.S., Mbati, P., Namangala, B., et al., (2010). Loop-mediated isothermal amplification (LAMP) assays for detection of Theileria parva infections targeting the PIM and p150 genes. Int. J. Parasitol. 40, 55–61.

Thuy, N.T., Goto, Y., Lun, Z.R., Kawazu, S. and Inoue, N. (2012). Tandem repeat protein as potential diagnostic antigen for Trypanosoma evansi infection. Parsitol. Res., 110: 733-739.

Torioni de Echaide, S., Florencia Bono, M., Lugaresi, C., Aguirre, N., Mangold, A., Moretta, R., Farber, M., Mondillo, C. (2005). Detection of antibodies against Anaplasma marginale in milk using a recombinant MSP5 indirect ELISA. Vet. Microbiol. 106, 287–292.

Torioni de Echaide, S., Knowles, D.P., McGuire, T.C., Palmer, G.H., Suarez, C.E., McElwain, T.F., (1998). Detection of cattle naturally infected with Anaplasma marginale in a region of endemicity by nested PCR and a competitive enzyme linked immunosorbent assay using recombinant major surface protein 5. J. Clin. Microbiol. 36, 777–782.

Vanlalhmuaka, Bansal, G.C., Saravanan, B.C., Rao, J.R. and Ray, D.D. (2010). Evaluation of pre-erythrocytic stage recombinant proteins of Theileria annulata for early diagnosis of bovine tropical theileriosis in Indian cattle. Indian J. Anim. Sci., 80(9): 822-825.

Vatansever, Z. and Nalbantoglu, S. (2002). Detection of cattle infected with Theileria annulata in fields by nested PCR, IFAT and microscopic examination of blood smears. Turk. J. Vet. Anim. Sci., 26: 1465-1469.

Verloo, D.; Magnus, E.; Buscher, P. (2001). General Expression of RoTat 1.2 Variable Antigen Type in Trypanosoma evansi Isolates from Different Origin. Vet. Parasitol., 97, 185–191.

Wagner, G.; Cruz, D.; Holman, P.; Waghela, S.; Perrone, J.; Shompole, S.; Rurangirwa, F. (1992). Non-immunologic methods of diagnosis of babesiosis. Mem. Inst. Oswaldo Cruz., 87, 193–199.

Wang, L.X., He, L., Fang, R., Song, Q.Q., Tu, P., Jenkins, A., et al., (2010). Loop-mediated isothermal amplification (LAMP) assay for detection of Theileria sergenti infection targeting the p33 gene. Vet. Parasitol. 171, 159–162.

Xie, J., Liu, G., Tian, Z., Luo, J., (2013). Development of loop-mediated isothermal amplification (LAMP) for detection of Theileria equi. Acta Trop. 127, 245–250.

Yadav, S.C., Kumar, R., Kumar, V., Jaideep, K.R., Gupta, A.K., Bera, B.C. and Tatu, U. (2013). Identification of immunodominant antigens of Trypanosoma evansi for detection of chronic trypanosomosis using experimentally infected equines. Res. Vet. Sci., 95(2): 522-528.

Yang, Y., Mao, Y., Kelly, P., Yang, Z., Luan, L., Zhang, J., et al., (2014). A pan-Theileria FRET-qPCR survey for Theileria spp. in ruminants from nine provinces of China. Parasit. Vectors 7, 413.

Yang, Y.; Li, Q.; Wang, S.; Chen, X.; Du, A., (2016). Rapid and sensitive detection of Babesia bovis and Babesia bigemina by loop-mediated isothermal amplification combined with a lateral flow dipstick. Vet. Parasitol., 30, 71–76.

Zaeemi, M., Haddadzadeh, H., Khazraiinia, P., Kazemi, B., Bandehpour, M., (2011). Identification of different Theileria species (Theileria lestoquardi, Theileria ovis, and Theileria annulata) in naturally infected sheep using nested PCR-RFLP. Parasitol. Res. 108, 837–843.

Zintl, A.; Mulcahy, G.; Skerrett, H.E.; Taylor, S.M.; Gray, J.S. (2003). Babesia divergens, a bovine blood parasite of veterinary and zoonotic importance. Clinical microbiology reviews, 16, (4), 622-636.

# 7

# Resistance to Anti-Protozoal With Special Emphasis on Haemoprotozoa of Dairy Animals

***Atul Prakash, S. Simran Kour, Shikha Verma and Anjali Yadav***

*Department of Veterinary Pharmacology and Toxicology, College of Veterinary Science and Animal Husbandry, U.P. Pt. Deen Dayal Upadhyaya Pashu Chikitsa Vigyan Vishwavidyalaya Evam Go Anusandhan Sansthan Mathura, Uttar Pradesh*

Livestock has been essential for Indian agriculture since prehistoric times. Livestock is crucial for tripling farmers' revenue, for bovines—particularly cattle and buffaloes—play a crucial role in the economy. India has the largest number of livestock owners, with a wide variety of livestock and poultry breeds that are essential to the socioeconomic advancement of rural communities. The production of consumables and maintaining the country's food security are inextricably related to the livestock and agricultural sectors. Numerous illnesses have a detrimental effect on the health and productivity of livestock and are highly significant economically. Livestock illnesses have negative effects on producers, costing them money in upkeep, resources, and production.

Protozoal infections are a major contributor to the global burden of infectious diseases and have a profound effect on health, society, and the economy. Nearly one-sixth of the world's population is at risk of dying from serious diseases like malaria (*Plasmodium* spp.), African sleeping sickness (*Trypanosoma brucei*), Chagas' disease (*Trypanosoma cruzi*) and various forms of cutaneous and visceral leishmaniasis (*Leishmania* spp.). Although the burden of protozoal diseases primarily affects tropical and subtropical regions, environmental changes and ecological modifications brought about by both natural and man-made factors have had and are likely to continue to have a significant impact on the emergence and spread of these infections in high-income nations.

Cattle are frequently infected with hemoprotozoan diseases, which have a severe impact on the livestock sector and constitute a serious danger to the global dairy industry. A significant economic factor in Asia, the majority of hemoprotozoan parasites are spread by ticks and have long posed a strong threat to the survival of exotic and crossbred cattle in India. The hot, muggy weather is ideal for the growth and survival of possible vectors like flies and ticks, and it continuously infects vulnerable animals. The three main tick-borne hemoprotozoan diseases that affect crossbred cattle in tropical and sub-tropical areas of the world are theileriosis, babesiosis, and anaplasmosis.

An estimated US $800 million is lost each year in India as a result of tropical theileriosis alone. These hemoprotozoan illnesses have a major negative economic impact on cow production in the form of mortality, decreased milk yield, and decreased draft power when proper control measures are not implemented. There have been reports of hemoprotozoan infections in India from various geographical areas. In cross-bred cattle, theileriosis incidence was 27.2%, with the maximum prevalence rate of 45.4% occurring during the rainy season in the Dehradun district of Uttarakhand, India. Cross-bred cattle in Gujarat's Anand area had overall rates of hemoprotozoan illnesses, including theileriosis (37%), babesiosis (10.41%), and anaplasmosis (2.82%). According to reports, the prevalence of theileriosis and babesiosis in crossbred cattle in Northern Kerala is 16% and 0.6%, respectively. There has been a documented theileriosis outbreak in cattle from Punjab, with a mortality rate of 4.86%.

The significant impact of protozoan infections has been compounded by the absence of safe, reasonably priced medications and effective vaccinations for the prevention and treatment of these illnesses. Unfortunately, the emergence of parasite drug resistance is posing a growing danger to the effectiveness of currently available medications.

Babesiosis is a tick-borne disease caused by protozoan parasites of the *Babesia* genus. It affects a variety of animals, including cattle, dogs, horses, and even wildlife such as deer. The parasites infect red blood cells, leading to haemolysis (destruction of red blood cells), anaemia, and other clinical signs. Bovine parasitic diseases, such as babesiosis, an infectious tick-borne hemoprotozoal disease brought on by *Babesia bigemina* and *Babesia bovis*, can significantly impair the health of the animal and result in significant financial losses. It is one of the most common and expensive tick-borne diseases (TBDs) affecting cattle globally.

Bovids are also impacted by *B. orientalis*, *B. ovata*, *B. major*, *B. motasi* and *B. venatorum* among other babesia species. Tristeza, Texas fever, redwater fever, tick fever, bovine babesiosis, and piroplasmosis are some other names for the illness. Efforts are being made to avoid and control it because it is prevalent in tropical and sub-tropical regions of the world and has a comparatively high morbidity and fatality rate. Ticks mechanically spread the disease to cows, primarily through the species *Boophilus* and *Hyalomma* spp. Cattle contract the infection when an infected tick injects the parasite's sporozoite stage into their blood stream during a blood meal. It has significant economic significance because the disease costs India's livestock industry about $57.2 million USD a year. According to a case study done in 2012 on an organized farm in Meghalaya, a milch cross-bred cow contracted *B. bigemina*, resulting in a loss of milk of 51.6 liters and an economic loss of 1032 rupees (12.92 US dollars) from a 30-day drop in production.

## Babesiosis

### 1. Cattle (Bovine Babesiosis)

- **Causative Agents:** The primary species that cause babesiosis in cattle are *Babesia bovis* and *Babesia bigemina.*
- **Transmission:** Mainly transmitted by ticks of the *Rhipicephalus* genus, such as the brown cattle tick (*Rhipicephalus microplus*).
- **Clinical Signs:** Symptoms include fever, weakness, anaemia, jaundice, red or dark-coloured urine (haemoglobinuria), and weight loss. In severe cases, it can be fatal.

### 2. Dogs (Canine Babesiosis)

- **Causative Agents:** The main species affecting dogs are *Babesia canis* and *Babesia gibsoni*. *Babesia vogeli* is another species known to infect dogs.
- **Transmission:** Transmitted by ticks such as *Rhipicephalus sanguineus* (brown dog tick) and through blood transfusions or dog fights.
- **Clinical Signs:** Dogs may exhibit fever, lethargy, pale mucous membranes (due to anemia), jaundice, red urine, and enlarged spleen or liver. Severe cases can lead to multi-organ failure and death.

### 3. Horses (Equine Babesiosis/Piroplasmosis)

- **Causative Agents:** In horses, the disease is often referred to as equine piroplasmosis and is caused by *Babesia caballi* and *Theileria equi* (a closely related parasite).

- **Transmission:** Spread by ticks like *Dermacentor* spp., *Rhipicephalus* spp., and *Amblyomma* spp. It can also be transmitted through contaminated needles and blood transfusions.
- **Clinical Signs:** Horses can develop fever, anemia, jaundice, weight loss, and in chronic cases, poor performance and lethargy.

**4. Wildlife**

- **Deer:** *Babesia odocoilei* is a species that infects white-tailed deer and other cervids. Though often asymptomatic, it can sometimes cause clinical disease, particularly in stressed or immunocompromised animals.
- **Other Wild Animals:** Babesiosis has been reported in wildlife species such as foxes, raccoons, and wolves, often with subclinical infections.
- **Common Drugs:**
    - **Imidocarb dipropionate:** This is one of the most commonly used drugs for treating babesiosis in animals, especially cattle, dogs, and horses. It helps in eliminating the *Babesia* parasites and providing some degree of protection against re-infection.
    - **Diminazene aceturate:** Frequently used for bovine babesiosis and canine cases. It is effective against several species of *Babesia* but requires careful dosing due to the potential for toxicity.
    - **Atovaquone and azithromycin:** This combination is used in dogs to treat infections caused by *Babesia gibsoni*. Atovaquone inhibits the parasite's mitochondrial electron transport, while azithromycin has anti-protozoal and anti-inflammatory effects.
- **Supportive Therapy:** In cases of severe anaemia, blood transfusions and supportive care may be necessary.

**Diagnosis**

- **Blood Smear:** Microscopic examination of stained blood smears can reveal the presence of *Babesia* parasites within red blood cells.
- **Serological Tests:** Various tests, including indirect fluorescent antibody tests (IFAT) and enzyme-linked immunosorbent assays (ELISA), can detect antibodies against *Babesia* species.
- **PCR (Polymerase Chain Reaction):** A sensitive method for detecting *Babesia* DNA in blood samples, allowing for more accurate identification of the species involved

- **Biosecurity Practices:**
  - Quarantine and testing of new animals before introducing them to existing herds can help prevent the introduction of *Babesia* into a population.
- **Vaccination:**
  - Vaccines are available for certain *Babesia* species in cattle, particularly for *B. bovis*, and can help reduce disease incidence.

## Zoonotic Potential

Babesiosis is primarily an animal disease, but *Babesia microti* (a species primarily affecting rodents) can infect humans, causing human babesiosis. However, the strains affecting livestock (like *B. bovis* and *B. bigemina*) are not zoonotic.

## Trypanosomiasis

Trypanosomiasis, also known as "sleeping sickness" in humans and "surra" in animals, is a parasitic disease caused by protozoan parasites of the *Trypanosoma* genus. It affects a wide range of animals, including livestock, pets, and wildlife. The disease is transmitted primarily through the bite of infected tsetse flies, but other biting insects, such as horseflies, can also transmit certain species. Trypanosomiasis remains a major veterinary and public health issue in tropical and subtropical regions, particularly in Africa, where it significantly impacts livestock health, agricultural productivity, and rural economies.

### 1. Trypanosomiasis in Cattle (Nagana)

- **Causative Agents:** In cattle, the main species responsible are *Trypanosoma brucei*, *Trypanosoma congolense*, and *Trypanosoma vivax*.
- **Transmission:** Transmitted mainly by tsetse flies (*Glossina* spp.) in sub-Saharan Africa. Mechanical transmission by biting flies (e.g., Tabanidae) can also occur, particularly for *T. vivax*.
- **Clinical Signs:** Cattle with trypanosomiasis may exhibit fever, lethargy, anemia, weight loss, swollen lymph nodes, reduced milk production, and abortion. Chronic cases can result in death if untreated.

### 2. Trypanosomiasis in Horses (Surra)

- **Causative Agent:** In horses, *Trypanosoma evansi* is the primary species causing surra.

- **Transmission:** Transmitted through biting flies such as Tabanids (horseflies), *Stomoxys* (stable flies), and even ticks.
- **Clinical Signs:** Horses can present with fever, anemia, edema (especially in the legs and belly), weakness, emaciation, and nervous symptoms like incoordination. It can be fatal without treatment.

**3. Trypanosomiasis in Dogs and Cats**

- **Causative Agents:** Dogs can be infected by *Trypanosoma cruzi*, which causes Chagas disease (common in the Americas), and *Trypanosoma evansi* (causing surra in regions like Asia and Africa).
- **Transmission:** *T. cruzi* is primarily spread through contact with the feces of infected triatomine bugs (kissing bugs), while *T. evansi* is spread by biting flies.
- **Clinical Signs in Dogs:** Symptoms include fever, lethargy, swollen lymph nodes, heart disease (myocarditis), and neurological signs. In advanced cases, it can lead to heart failure.

**4. Trypanosomiasis in Camels and Other Livestock**

- **Causative Agents:** Camels are particularly susceptible to *Trypanosoma evansi* (surra), which can also infect other livestock such as goats, sheep, and pigs.
- **Transmission:** Biting flies, including horseflies and stable flies, are the primary vectors.
- **Clinical Signs in Camels:** Symptoms include fever, progressive weight loss, anemia, swelling of the lower body, and occasional nervous symptoms. If untreated, the disease can be fatal.

**5. Wildlife and Trypanosomiasis**

- Wildlife species such as antelope, buffalo, and wild dogs can be reservoirs for *Trypanosoma* species, making eradication challenging. Some species exhibit resistance or tolerance to infection, serving as asymptomatic carriers.
- **Common Drugs**
    - **Diminazene aceturate:** Widely used in veterinary practice for treating trypanosomiasis in cattle, horses, camels, and dogs. It is effective against *Trypanosoma* species but has a narrow safety margin.

  - **Suramin:** Used for the treatment of trypanosomiasis in horses and camels, particularly for *Trypanosoma evansi* infections. It has a long-acting effect but can cause side effects in some animals.
  - **Isometamidium chloride:** This drug is used for both treatment and prevention in cattle. It has a prolonged action and protect against reinfection.
  - **Melarsomine dihydrochloride:** Sometimes used for canine infections, especially when other drugs are ineffective.
- **Supportive Care:** Fluid therapy and nutritional support are often provided alongside drug treatment.

### Diagnosis

- **Blood Smear:** Microscopic examination of blood smears can detect trypomastigotes in the blood.
- **Serological Tests:** ELISA and other serological assays can be used to detect antibodies against *Trypanosoma* species.
- **Molecular Methods:** PCR assays can help confirm the presence of the parasite in blood or tissue samples.

### Prevention and Control

- **Vector Control:** Reducing the population of tsetse flies through traps, insecticides, and habitat management.
- **Cattle Management:** Regular screening of animals for infection and culling of infected animals.
- **Vaccination:** There is no effective vaccine against trypanosomiasis in livestock, but research is ongoing.
- **Good Husbandry Practices:** Maintaining good hygiene, proper nutrition, and reducing stress in animals can help improve their resistance to infections.

### Zoonotic Potential

While *Trypanosoma brucei* can infect humans, the primary concern is for domestic animals in endemic regions. In contrast, *Trypanosoma evansi* does not pose a direct risk to humans but can cause significant health issues in affected animals.

## Leishmaniosis

Leishmaniosis is a parasitic disease caused by protozoan parasites of the *Leishmania* genus. It affects various animals, including dogs, cats, rodents, and wildlife, and can also be transmitted to humans (zoonotic disease). The parasites are transmitted through the bites of infected female sandflies, primarily of the *Phlebotomus* and *Lutzomyia* genera, depending on the geographic region. Leishmaniosis is an important zoonotic disease that affects animal health, especially in tropical and subtropical regions, southern Europe, and parts of Latin America. Early diagnosis and control strategies focused on sandfly vector management, reservoir host control, and preventive treatments are crucial in managing this disease.

### 1. Leishmaniosis in Dogs (Canine Leishmaniosis)

- **Causative Agent:** The primary species causing disease in dogs is *Leishmania infantum* (also known as *Leishmania chagasi* in Latin America).
- **Transmission:** The main mode of transmission is through the bite of infected sandflies. In some cases, transmission can occur through blood transfusions, vertical transmission (from mother to puppies), or dog bites.
- **Clinical Forms:**
  - **Visceral Leishmaniosis:** Affects internal organs such as the liver, spleen, lymph nodes, and bone marrow.
- **Cutaneous Leishmaniosis:** Leads to skin lesions, ulcers, and alopecia (hair loss), often around the eyes, ears, and nose.
- **Clinical Signs:** Dogs may exhibit symptoms such as weight loss, lethargy, enlarged lymph nodes, skin lesions, excessive nail growth, bleeding from the nose, and kidney dysfunction. Some dogs remain asymptomatic but still act as reservoirs for the parasite.

### 2. Leishmaniosis in Cats (Feline Leishmaniosis)

- **Causative Agent:** *Leishmania infantum* is also responsible for leishmaniosis in cats, though the disease is less common and usually less severe than in dogs.
- **Transmission:** Similar to dogs, transmission occurs through the bites of infected sandflies.

- **Clinical Signs:** Infected cats may present with skin lesions, nodules, ulcers, and, less commonly, systemic signs such as weight loss, fever, or lymph node enlargement.

**3. Leishmaniosis in Horses and Other Livestock**

- **Horses:** *Leishmania* infection in horses is uncommon but can cause cutaneous leishmaniosis, as nodules or ulcerated skin lesions, typically on the head, ears, or neck.
- **Other Livestock:** Cattle, goats, and sheep are rarely affected by *Leishmania* species and, if infected, usually show mild or asymptomatic cases.

**4. Leishmaniosis in Wildlife**

- **Reservoir Hosts:** Wild animals, such as foxes, rodents, and wild canids, can act as reservoirs for *Leishmania* parasites, helping maintain the transmission cycle.
- **Wild Canids:** Foxes and other wild canids often serve as important reservoirs for *Leishmania infantum*, especially in areas where the disease is endemic.
- **Rodents:** Some rodent species can harbor *Leishmania* and are implicated in the maintenance of the transmission cycle, particularly in regions with endemic cutaneous leishmaniosis.
- **Common Drugs:**
    - **Meglumine antimoniate:** This antimonial compound is used as a first-line treatment for canine leishmaniosis. It works by inhibiting the metabolic processes of the *Leishmania* parasite.
    - **Miltefosine:** An oral medication used to treat leishmaniosis in dogs. It disrupts parasite membranes and is effective against both cutaneous and visceral forms.
    - **Allopurinol:** Often used as a maintenance therapy to suppress the replication of *Leishmania* in dogs. It helps in preventing relapse but does not eliminate the parasite completely.

**Amphotericin B:** This antifungal agent is used as a second-line treatment for severe or refractory cases of canine leishmaniosis.

**Supportive Care:** Includes dietary management, treatment of concurrent infections, and monitoring for kidney damage (a common complication).

**Diagnosis**

- **Clinical Signs:** Diagnosis often starts with a clinical examination and history of exposure to sandfly habitats.
- **Blood Tests:** Serological tests can detect antibodies against *Leishmania.*
- **Bone Marrow or Spleen Aspirate:** Microscopic examination can reveal the presence of *Leishmania* amastigotes within macrophages.

**PCR (Polymerase Chain Reaction):** A sensitive method to detect *Leishmania* DNA in blood, tissue samples, or aspirates.

• **Visceral Leishmaniasis**

- **Antimonial compounds (e.g., sodium stibogluconate):** Historically the mainstay of treatment.
- **Allopurinol:** Often used in combination with other treatments for chronic cases.
- **Miltefosine:** An oral treatment effective against *Leishmania.*
- **Amphotericin B:** An alternative for severe cases

• **Cutaneous Leishmaniasis**

- Treatment may include topical agents, such as paromomycin or local cryotherapy, depending on the species and severity of lesions.
- Systemic treatment may be required for extensive or refractory cases.

**Prevention and Control**

- **Vector Control:** Reducing exposure to sandflies through the use of insecticides, insect repellents, and environmental management (removing breeding sites).
- **Vaccination:** There are vaccines available in some regions (e.g., Leishmune) that can help reduce the incidence of visceral leishmaniasis in dogs.
- **Limit Outdoor Exposure:** Keeping dogs indoors during peak sandfly activity (dusk and dawn) can reduce the risk of transmission.
- **Regular Veterinary Care:** Routine health checks can help detect and

**Zoonotic Potential**

**Visceral Leishmaniasis** is a significant zoonotic disease, with infected dogs acting as a reservoir for *Leishmania infantum.* Humans can become infected through sandfly bites or, in rare cases, through direct contact with infected dogs.

## Anaplasmosis

Anaplasmosis is a tick-borne disease caused by bacteria from the genus *Anaplasma*. It primarily affects livestock such as cattle, sheep, and goats, but can also infect other animals, including dogs, horses, and wildlife. The disease is characterized by the infection and destruction of red blood cells, leading to symptoms associated with anaemia. Anaplasmosis is a significant concern in animal health, particularly for cattle in tropical and subtropical regions. Preventive measures and early diagnosis are essential to managing the disease and minimizing its impact on livestock productivity.

### 1. Anaplasmosis in Cattle (Bovine Anaplasmosis)

- **Causative Agent:** The main pathogen responsible is *Anaplasma marginale*, though *Anaplasma centrale* can also infect cattle.
- **Transmission:** Transmitted mainly through tick bites, especially from species like *Dermacentor*, *Rhipicephalus*, and *Ixodes*. It can also spread through mechanical transmission (contaminated needles, dehorning instruments, or biting flies).
- **Clinical Signs:** Symptoms range from mild to severe and include fever, lethargy, pale or yellowish mucous membranes (jaundice), anemia, rapid heart rate, weight loss, decreased milk production, and, in severe cases, death. Young cattle are usually less severely affected than older animals.

### 2. Anaplasmosis in Sheep and Goats (Ovine and Caprine Anaplasmosis)

- **Causative Agent:** In small ruminants, *Anaplasma ovis* is the primary pathogen.
- **Transmission:** Similar to cattle, transmission occurs through tick bites, mechanical transmission, or biting flies.
- **Clinical Signs:** The disease is often milder in sheep and goats compared to cattle. Symptoms include fever, lethargy, pale mucous membranes, decreased appetite, and weight loss. In severe cases, animals may show signs of respiratory distress or collapse.

### 3. Anaplasmosis in Dogs (Canine Anaplasmosis)

- **Causative Agents:** In dogs, *Anaplasma phagocytophilum* and *Anaplasma platys* are the main pathogens. *A. phagocytophilum* causes granulocytic anaplasmosis, while *A. platys* causes thrombocytopenia (low platelet count).

- **Transmission:** Spread primarily by tick bites, especially from *Ixodes* species (black-legged tick or deer tick) for *A. phagocytophilum* and *Rhipicephalus sanguineus* (brown dog tick) for *A. platys*.
- **Clinical Signs:** Symptoms may include fever, lethargy, joint pain, lameness, loss of appetite, and, in the case of *A. platys*, bleeding disorders due to low platelets. In some cases, dogs may show no symptoms (subclinical infection).

### 4. Anaplasmosis in Horses (Equine Granulocytic Anaplasmosis)

- **Causative Agent:** *Anaplasma phagocytophilum* is the species affecting horses.
- **Transmission:** Transmitted by *Ixodes* ticks, which are also vectors for Lyme disease.
- **Clinical Signs:** Horses may develop fever, depression, limb edema, jaundice, reluctance to move, ataxia, and petechiae (small hemorrhages). Some horses recover without treatment, while others may experience severe symptoms.

### 5. Anaplasmosis in Wildlife

- **Wild Ruminants:** Deer and other wild ruminants can act as reservoirs for *Anaplasma* species, contributing to the spread of the disease to domestic animals.
- **Rodents and Small Mammals:** These animals may also serve as reservoirs for *Anaplasma phagocytophilum*, facilitating transmission in certain regions.

## Theileriosis

Theileriosis is a tick-borne disease caused by protozoan parasites of the genus *Theileria*. It primarily affects cattle but can also infect other livestock species, such as sheep and goats, as well as some wild animals. The disease can lead to significant economic losses in the livestock industry due to decreased productivity and increased veterinary costs.

### 1. Etiology and Species Affected

- **Theileria parva:** The causative agent of East Coast fever in cattle, primarily found in eastern and southern Africa.

- **Theileria annulata:** Associated with tropical theileriosis, affecting cattle in Africa, the Middle East, and parts of Asia.
- **Other Species:** Other *Theileria* species can also infect small ruminants and wildlife, though *T. parva* and *T. annulata* are the most economically significant.

**2. Transmission**

- **Vector-borne Transmission:** The primary mode of transmission is through the bite of infected ticks, primarily of the *Rhipicephalus* (formerly *Boophilus*) genus, which transmit the parasites from infected animals to healthy ones.
- **Direct Contact:** Rarely, transmission can occur through direct contact with infected blood or tissues.

**3. Clinical Signs**

The clinical presentation of theileriosis can vary based on the species involved and the host's immune response but commonly includes:

- **Acute Theileriosis (East Coast Fever):**
    - Fever (often high)
    - Lethargy and weakness
    - Anorexia (loss of appetite)
    - Swelling of lymph nodes (lymphadenopathy)
    - Coughing and respiratory distress (occasionally)
    - Neurological signs (in severe cases)
- **Chronic Theileriosis (Tropical Theileriosis):**
    - Anemia (often severe)
    - Weight loss
    - Pale mucous membranes
    - Icterus (jaundice)
    - Weakness

**4. Diagnosis**

- **Clinical Signs:** Diagnosis often begins with a clinical examination and history of exposure to tick-infested areas.

- **Blood Smear:** Microscopic examination of blood can reveal the presence of *Theileria* parasites in red blood cells. *Theileria* species can be identified based on their morphology.
- **PCR (Polymerase Chain Reaction):** A more sensitive method for detecting *Theileria* DNA in blood samples.
- **Serological Tests:** Can help identify antibodies against *Theileria* species, aiding in diagnosis.

### 5. Treatment

- **Antimicrobial Therapy:**
    - **Imidocarb dipropionate:** Commonly used for treating theileriosis.
    - **Oxytetracycline:** Effective against *Theileria* and often used in combination therapy.
    - **Other Antiparasitic Drugs:** May be employed in specific cases, depending on the species and severity of infection.
- **Supportive Care:** Providing fluids, nutritional support, and managing complications like anemia and dehydration is critical for recovery.

### 6. Prevention and Control

- **Vector Control**
    - Regular use of tick preventives, including acaricides, can help reduce tick populations and minimize exposure.
    - Environmental management to reduce tick habitats.
- **Vaccination:** In some regions, vaccines are available to protect against specific *Theileria* infections, such as *T. parva*.
- **Monitoring and Health Checks:** Routine veterinary care and monitoring of livestock for early signs of illness can aid in prevention and control.

### 7. Zoonotic Potential

There is currently no significant evidence to suggest that *Theileria* species pose a zoonotic risk to humans. The primary concern is for livestock health.

## Hepatozoonosis

Hepatozoonosis is a disease caused by protozoan parasites of the genus *Hepatozoon*, affecting various animal species, particularly dogs however, it can affect a variety of animals, including cattle, dogs, and other mammals. The most notable species is *Hepatozoon canis*, which primarily affects dogs, while *Hepatozoon americanum* is found in the America and is also a significant pathogen in dogs.

### 1. Etiology and Species Affected

- **Hepatozoon canis:** Primarily affects dogs, causing a disease known as canine hepatozoonosis. It is transmitted by the brown dog tick (*Rhipicephalus sanguineus*).
- **Hepatozoon americanum:** Also affects dogs and is transmitted by the *Amblyomma maculatum* (gulf coast tick). This species is associated with severe disease.
- Hepatozoon parasites can also infect other mammals, including some wild canids and rodents.

### 2. Transmission

- **Vector-borne Transmission:** The primary mode of transmission is through the ingestion of an infected tick. Unlike other vector-borne diseases, *Hepatozoon* is not transmitted through the bite of an infected tick but rather through the ingestion of the tick during grooming.
- **Direct Contact:** Rarely, infection can occur through contact with infected tissues or blood.

### 3. Clinical Signs

- **Acute Phase:** Fever, Lethargy and weakness, Anorexia, Muscle pain or stiffness (often observed as reluctance to move)
  - Diarrhea
  - Weight loss
  - Mild cough (occasionally)
- **Chronic Phase:**
  - Weight loss
  - Anemia
  - Lethargy
  - Persistent fever
  - Muscle atrophy
  - Potential organ involvement (such as liver and spleen enlargement)

### 4. Diagnosis

- **Blood Smear:** Microscopic examination of blood or tissue samples can reveal the presence of *Hepatozoon* gametocytes within white blood cells (neutrophils).
- **Serological Tests:** Various serological assays can detect antibodies against *Hepatozoon* species.
- **PCR (Polymerase Chain Reaction):** A sensitive method to identify *Hepatozoon* DNA in blood, muscle tissue, or biopsies.
- **Imaging:** Radiographs or ultrasound may reveal muscle atrophy or organ enlargement.

### 5. Treatment

- **Antimicrobial Therapy:**
    - **Tetracyclines (e.g., doxycycline):** Commonly used to manage acute infections.
    - **Clindamycin:** May be used as an alternative.
- **Supportive Care:** Management of clinical signs, including hydration and nutrition, is essential. Pain management may be necessary for muscle pain or discomfort.
- **Long-term Treatment:** In cases of chronic infection, prolonged treatment may be needed, including a combination of medications.

### 6. Prevention and Control

- **Vector Control:** Reducing tick exposure is crucial. This includes regular use of tick preventives, such as topical or oral acaricides.
- **Environment Management:** Maintaining clean living areas and regularly checking for ticks can help reduce the risk of infection.
- **Regular Veterinary Care:** Routine health checks can help with early detection and management of infections.

### 7. Zoonotic Potential

There is no significant evidence suggesting that *Hepatozoon* species pose a zoonotic risk to humans. However, as with many parasitic infections, maintaining good hygiene and health practices around pets is advisable.

## Mechanisms of resistance development

- **Intrinsic resistance**: Parasites evolve to change their structure or components to survive antiprotozoal drugs.
- **Acquired resistance**: Protozoans can acquire resistance through a genetic mutation or by transfer of DNA from a resistant parasite.
- **Enzymatic degradation**: Protozoans may produce enzymes that inactivate antiprotozoal drugs.
- **Target protection**: A target protection protein binds to the antiprotozoal drug target.
- **Active efflux**: Transmembrane efflux pumps remove antiparasitic drugs from protozoal cells.
- **Reduced drug penetration**: Change in membrane permeability to antiprotozoal drugs.
- **Horizontal gene transfer**: Sharing genetic components with other hemoprotozoan, which can lead to the spread of resistance.
- **Overexpression of ABC transporters:** The overexpression of membrane-bound ATP-binding cassette (ABC) transporters on the surface of *Leishmania* parasites can contribute to antimonial resistance.
- **Point mutations**: Point mutations in dihydrofolate reductase and dihydropteroate synthase can cause resistance to antifolates.
- **High treatment frequency**: Frequent treatment can lead to resistance more strongly than less frequent dosing regimens.
- **Using the same drug over many years**: Resistance can develop even when only two or three treatments are given annually, especially when the same drug is used over many years.

## Factors Involved in the Spread of Resistance

The ease with which a certain drug can select resistant individual microorganisms and the potential for resistance to spread in a population, and hence the significance to public health, are two crucial factors to take into account when analyzing the significance of a drug resistance problem. First, **the volume** (dose and frequency) of drug use, **the likelihood that a drug-sensitive infection** will become resistant upon infection, **the length of time** an individual is infected, **the fitness costs** (division rate and transmissibility) for the pathogen incurred by being resistant in the absence of drugs, and the **extent to which compensatory mechanisms develop** to offset these fitness costs are the main measurable parameters that govern the spread of drug-resistant genotypes through a population of microorganisms.

## Host, Parasite and Drug resistance

Although the burden of protozoal diseases primarily affects tropical and subtropical regions, environmental changes and ecological modifications brought about by both natural and man-made factors have had and are likely to continue to have a significant impact on the emergence and spread of these infections in high-income nations.

The significant impact of human protozoan infections has been compounded by the absence of safe, reasonably priced medications and effective vaccinations for the prevention and treatment of these illnesses. Unfortunately, the emergence of parasite drug resistance is posing a growing danger to the effectiveness of currently available medications. Global research is driven by the need for novel antiprotozoal medications, which calls for creative approaches to guarantee a sustained lead compound discovery.

Treatment of infectious disorders is hampered by the development of medication resistance in pathogens, which include bacteria, protozoa, and fungus. Through a variety of mechanisms, including genetic alterations in the target sites, decreased drug absorption and greater drug efflux, and metabolic regulation, protozoan parasites have become resistant to a number of antiprotozoal treatments over the past few decades. Treatment of clinical cases is significantly impacted by the rise of drug-resistant parasites, which raises morbidity and mortality.

## Antibabesial Drug Resistance

Intraerythrocytic parasites belonging to the genus *Babesia* spp. are the cause of the infectious illness babesiosis. There are around 100 species of Babesia known to exist. *Babesia bigemina, B. divergens*, and *B. bovis* for bovine are the most prominent species. Clinical signs such as fever, hemolytic anemia, anorexia, hemoglobinuria, and emaciation are caused by parasites replicating in the red blood cells (RBCs) of their mammalian hosts. The severe infection phase frequently leads to mortality. There are currently few therapy options for babesiosis. For example, diminazene aceturate and imidocarb dipropionate are used to treat animal babesiosis.

It is generally known that intraerythrocytic apicomplexan parasites, such as Babesia species, can develop treatment resistance. Babesia microti-caused human babesiosis is best treated with a combination therapy of atovaquone and azithromycin; however, strains of *B. microti* that are resistant to both medications have recently surfaced. Furthermore, atovaquone medication causes *Babesia gibsoni* in dogs to acquire resistance, according to a prior study. Point mutations that cause amino acid substitution in cytochrome b, the molecular target of atovaquone, are proposed as a potential mechanism of atovaquone resistance.

An antibabesial drug called diminazene aceturate (DA) is frequently used to treat animal babesiosis, which is brought on by a form of Babesia that is found all over the world. Only three species of *Babesia—B. bovis, B. bigemina, and B. divergens*—are known to cause severe clinical babesiosis, despite the fact that cattle are infected by several species of Babesia. Because the parasite-infected erythrocytes stick to the endothelial cells in the capillaries in internal organs like the brain and lungs, causing neurological and respiratory symptoms, *B. bovis* specifically produces the most severe type of bovine babesiosis.

The TbAT1 and TevAT1 genes, respectively, encode an adenosine transporter known as P2, which mediates the absorption of DA in *Trypanosoma brucei* and *T. equiperdium*. It has been suggested that DA-resistant strains' decreased P2 transporter activity causes low DA uptake into Trypanosoma, which lowers DA's effectiveness. Furthermore, elevated TeDR40 gene mRNA expression adds to *T. evansi* heightened resistance to DA. Research showed that DA treatment increased the expression of *B. bovis* mitochondrial (cob and cox3) and apicoplast (tufA and clpC) genes, whereas CF treatment decreased these genes. This may imply that temporally upregulated apicoplast and mitochondrial genes contribute to developing the unstable resistance in *B. bovis* to DA.

## Antileishmanial Drug Resistance

Leishmaniasis is a multifaceted tropical and subtropical illness, primarily caused by over 50 different species of parasitic protozoa in the genus Leishmania, 20 of which are harmful to humans. This illness is endemic in at least 98 countries, with a yearly incidence of one million new cases and 26–65 thousand deaths. There are over 90 species of female phlebotomine sandflies that spread the parasites amongst their mammalian hosts.

The illness manifests itself in various ways. (1) The most dangerous type of leishmaniasis, known as visceral leishmaniasis (VL) or kala-azar, is incurable if left untreated. Post-kala-azardermal leishmaniasis (PKDL) typically manifests six months to a year following the apparent resolution of VL. 3) The most prevalent type, cutaneous leishmaniasis (CL), results in skin lesions, primarily ulcers on exposed body parts, and leaves permanent scars. (4) Mucocutaneous leishmaniasis (MCL), which causes the throat, mouth, and nose mucous membranes to completely or partially degrade.

The parasite's life cycle manifests in two morphological forms: amastigotes in the macrophages of the mammalian host and promastigotes in the gut of the sand fly vectors. When metacyclic promastigotes are injected into the human body by a parasitized female sand fly, the life cycle enters the human stage. The parasite changes into an amastigote, a non-flagellated form, after being first phagocytosed by the host's macrophages of the skin. From there, parasites spread and infiltrate more macro.

## Resistance to Antimonials

### *Plausible mechanism of classical drugs resistance*

1) **Main mechanism of resistance includes**: First-line antimonial therapeutic modalities have been resistant owing to: efflux/sequestration of the active drug in association with trypanothione (TSH), and by increasing the levels of TSH and P-glycoprotein efflux pumps.
2) **Resistance against classical second-line therapeutic modalities has been induced due to**: modification of drug receptor binding site (sterol binding receptor), amplified biosynthesis of competitor substrate (polyamine) for drug transporter and active extrusion of the drug by efflux pumps.

Currently, the only effective treatment for all forms of leishmaniasis that produces satisfactory clinical and microbiological results is the pentavalent antimonials sodium stibogluconate (SSG) and meglumine antimoniate (MA). Since there are no available oral preparations, these medications can only be administered by injection and have serious side effects, such as pancreatitis, cardiac, and renal toxicity. Trypanothione reductase (TR), an enzyme thought to be essential for parasite survival in the host, is inhibited by both SSG and MA. In order to neutralize the reactive oxygen species generated by macrophages during the infection, the Leishmaniatryparedoxin/tryparedoxin peroxidase system (TXN/TXNPx) uses trypanothione, which is reduced by TR. Trypanothione is the primary detoxifying mechanism against oxidative damage in trypanosomatid parasites, as opposed to mammals, which use glutathione (GSH) as the essential component for redox defenses. It is widely acknowledged that pentavalent antimonials are prodrugs and that they are converted in vivo to the toxic and active trivalent antimonials Sb(III), which cause Leishmaniasis by causing apoptosis. Sb(V) is more likely to be reduced to Sb(III) in an acidic pH and at a slightly higher temperature. Both the parasite and macrophages may experience this decrease in antimonials. Leishmania's capacity to convert Sb(V) to Sb(III) varies depending on the stage. While promastigotes are unable to reduce Sb(V) to Sb(III), amastigotes are able to do so.

## Associated Mutations

Antimonial resistance developed slowly, indicating that multiple mutations might be needed to produce a resistance phenotype. Although the observed antimonial resistance can be explained by a number of in vitro mechanisms, it should be noted that in vitro responsiveness does not always equate to clinical resistance. The emergence of resistance can be explained by the following factors: geneamplification; inhibition of drug activation; inactivation of the active drug; and reduction of drug concentration within the parasite, either by decreasing drug uptake or by increasing drug efflux [70]. High levels of Sb(III) resistance are linked to overexpression of TXNPx and elevated intracellular thiol levels. An inhibition of Sb(V) activation and a decreased uptake of the active form Sb(III) by amastigotes in the thiol metabolism were confirmed in in vivo antimonial resistance. The genes aquaglyceroporin 1, γ-glutamylcysteine synthetase, and ornithine decarboxylase, which are involved in the uptake of Sb(III) and the metabolism of glutathione and trypathione, respectively, are expressed less during this process. The overexpression of the membrane-bound ATP-binding cassette (ABC) transporters on the surface of Leishmania parasites is another way that antimonial resistance occurs. This transport system contributes to the development of resistance by modulating the efflux and intracellular accumulation of different drugs. A can be facilitated by the ABC transporters ABCI4 and ABCG2.

For *Leishmania* to bind and internalize, host membrane cholesterol is necessary. In higher eukaryotes, cholesterol is a necessary membrane lipid that is essential to the dynamics, organization, and functionality of membrane constituents. The rate-limiting enzyme in the cholesterol biosynthesis pathway, HMG-CoA reductase, is competitively inhibited by statins like lovastatin. It has been demonstrated that lovastatin inhibits the proteins P-glycoproteinin L and MRP1. Donovani permits the buildup of antimony, which in turn inhibits the growth of Leishmania cells and macrophage infection, ultimately resulting in the death of the parasite. The statin class thus reverses Sb resistance.

In *Leishmania*, flavonoids are a class of naturally occurring inhibitors of P-glycoprotein and associated AB Ctransporters. Antimony drug resistance in *Leishmania* has been reversed using synthetic flavonoid dimers. *L. donovani* by boosting drug accumulation inside cells. It was discovered that the heat shock proteins (HSP70) play a part in antimony tolerance through functional cloning, which isolates drug resistance genes. Cells exposed to antimony and Sb(III)-resistant mutants were found to overexpress HSP70 proteins. Antimony resistance was higher in *Leishmania* species transfected with the HSP70 gene, presumably as a result of the cells' enhanced metal tolerance, which enabled the development of more precise and potent resistance mechanisms. HSP90 was also identified in recent research as a gene linked to the development of resistance in *Leishmania.* All things considered, antimonial resistance is a complex phenomenon. Several antimonial resistance mechanisms were found in clinical *Leishmania* isolates.

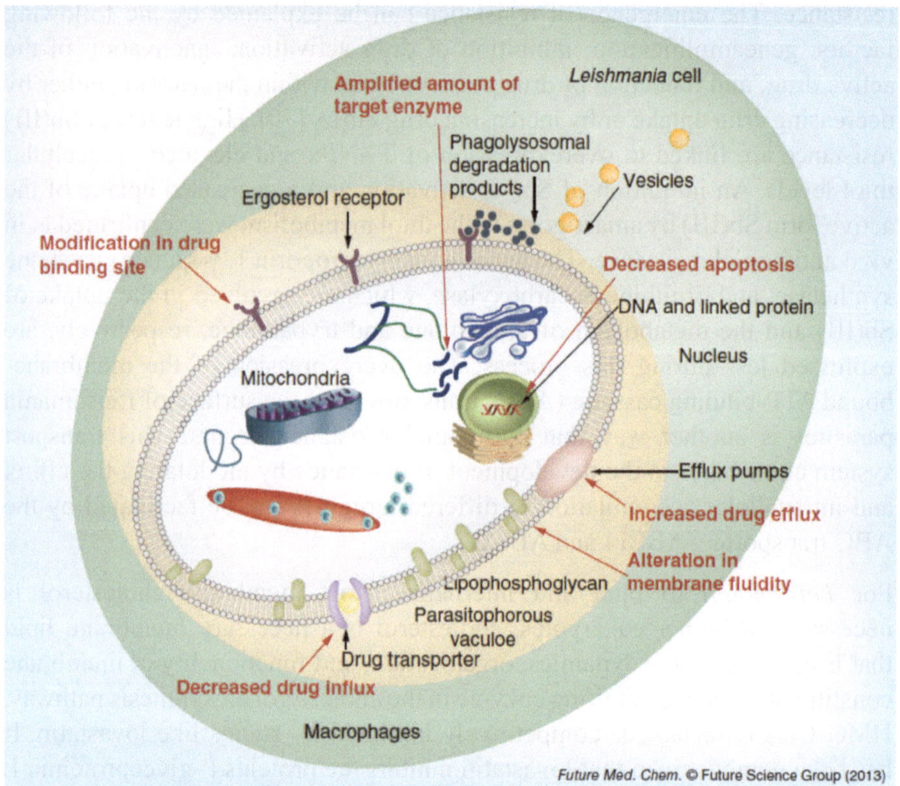


Mechanism of Drug resistance in a Leishmanial cell. Source: *Future Med. Chem.* (2013)

### *Resistance to Pentamidine*

In 1937, the aromatic diamidine pentamidine (PMD) was used to treat sleeping sickness. The first use of antimony in the treatment of VL cases with resistance was documented in 1949 in India. When L is the cause of systemic CL, PMD is administered. guyanensis as well as *L. panamensis*. However, the primary cause of this drug›s discontinuation in India in the 1990s was the emergence of PMD resistance as well as additional side effects, including hypoglycemia, hypotension, fever, myocarditis, and renal toxicity. Although the exact mode of action of PMD in Leishmania is unknown, some reports indicate that the drug interferes with the potential of the parasite›s inner membrane. The bloodstream form of L could potentially undergo apoptosis due to the accumulation of pentamidine in the mitochondria. Donovani increases the cytotoxicity of the drug by blocking the production of ROS, respiratory chain complexes I, II, and III, and cytosolic Ca2+ . Furthermore, DNA topoisomerases (TOPs), which are crucial for modifying DNA topology during transcription, replication, recombination, and repair, can also be targeted by PMD. *Leishmania* parasites' TOPI and TOPII enzymes differ significantly from corresponding human enzymes in terms of structure and biochemistry, and they play a crucial role in structuring the kinetoplast DNA network that is specific to these parasites. Research indicates that PMD exhibits selectivity towards *Leishmania* TOPII.

### *Associated mutations*

Mutations in a number of transporters have been implicated in pentamidine resistance in *Leishmania* parasites. Several species of *Leishmania* have been found to harbor ABC transporters, and several of these transporters have been thoroughly studied and linked to drug resistance. P-glycoprotein (PGP) and other members of the ABC transporters superfamily (ABCC7) include the pentamidine resistance protein 1 (PRP1). The transporter that gives trypanosomes their resistance to high concentrations of pentamidine and melarsoprol is aquaglyceroporin 2 (AQP2), a member of a family of surface channel protcins involved in the passive transport of water and small non-charged solutes across cell membranes. Research is necessary, but it's possible that pentamidine resistance in *Leishmania* parasites is also caused by an AQP2 mutation. It should come as no surprise that research has shown that the P-glycoprotein inhibitor and Ca2+ channel blocker rapamil can inhibit PMD efflux, causing PMD to accumulate in resistant parasites. Flavonoid dimers were synthesized to prevent pentamidine resistance in *Leishmania* parasites, and they showed a noticeably higher pentamidine resistance reversing activity in L. enriettii, as a result of the medication building up more in the mitochondria. These artificial flavonoids work as reversal agents to break the parasite *Leishmania's* resistance to PMD. Quinacrine and the same dimers had a synergistic effect on reversing.

## Resistance to Amphotericin B

The second-line medication for the treatment of VL is amphotericin B (AMB), a polyene antibiotic that was first isolated from the filamentous bacterium *Streptomyces nodosus*. In highly endemic areas like Bihar state in India, it is the most effective treatment for pentavalent antimonial refractive leishmaniasis. The National Program of Nepal currently recommends it for the treatment of kala-azar. Even though AMB is a very effective antileishmanial medication, it has serious side effects like acute nephrotoxicity, which necessitates hospitalization and close patient monitoring for the entire four-week course of treatment. The high price of AMB is yet another significant drawback. Liposomal AMB (LAMB), a lipid-associated formulation that has been developed to circumvent these limitations, has a longer plasma half-life and lower toxicity, enabling the administration of a single infusion. AMB formulations that are safer to take orally are being developed to treat leishmaniasis.

AMB may work by interacting with the sterols in the membrane, which causes the membrane to become disorganized and increases the permeability of protons and monovalent cations. AMB's auto-oxidation and subsequent production of free radicals may also have an impact on the cells. The production of reactive oxygen free radicals, oxidative effects, and ion movement may all be linked to the cell damage caused by AMB.

Because of the emergence of drug resistance to other treatments, amphotericin B is becoming a more significant treatment for leishmaniasis. Emergent resistance to AMB may pose an immediate threat because there aren't many alternative medications on the market. Therefore, it is crucial to identify the mechanisms through which AMB resistance can develop. This has resulted in the development of laboratory-derived AMB resistance in Leishmania spp.. Similarly, a relapse rate of 3–7% reported following liposomal amphotericin treatment indicates that resistance can develop for LAMB. However, despite this low risk, it is significant in the context of transmission dynamics because: a) relapse adds to the global pool of parasites in the host that are ready to be transmitted to the vector; b) relapse increases the risk of transmission in HIV-positive individuals who are not receiving antiretroviral therapy due to suppressive immunity, increased parasite burden, and lack of responsiveness to drug treatment; and c) patients with relapsed HIV co-infection may have parasite resistance to antileishmanial drugs, which could be a long-term reservoir resistant parasite or an increased risk of developing PKDL.

### *Associated Mutations*

As of right now, no effective resistance to AMB has been documented. In the lab, a number of tests have been created to predict the potential emergence of resistance. By applying increasing drug pressure, a number of promastigotes of AMB-resistant *Leishmania* spp. were chosen and examined. Several mutations were found when the biological characteristics of these resistant strains were contrasted with those of the parent strain of the wild type. A mutation in the sterolbiosynthesis enzyme, lanosterol 14α-demethylase (CYP51), was shown to play a part in a L. Mexican line. Two sterol biosynthesis enzymes, sterol

C24-methyltransferase (SMT), which adds the C24-methyl group to the ergosterolside chain, and sterol C5-desaturase (SC5D), which is necessary for the production of sterol 5(6)-7(8) doublebond conjugation, were also found to have genetic alterations in several AMB-resistant *Leishmania* lines.

The decreased AMB binding to the membrane as a result of a changed sterol profile (loss of function of the SMT gene) is the overall cause of the resistance. Following the membrane-bound MDR1's efflux of AMB, the intracellular AMB that remains auto-oxidizes and generates ROS. The thiol metabolic pathway's tryparedoxin cascade may counteract the harmful effects of these ROS. The *Leishmania* parasites' resistance to AMB may be caused by the cumulative effects of a modified membrane profile involving MDR1 and the tryparedoxin cascade.

## Resistance to Miltefosine

Miltefosine, also known as hexadecylphosphocholine (MT), is an alkyl phospholipid that was first created as an oral antitumor agent. In India, MT was authorized as the first oral treatment for VL in 2002. At the moment, MT is the first option for oral treatment in CL and is used to treat VL and CL diseases. Compared to antimonials, it is more accessible and less toxic. Hepatotoxicity and nephrotoxicity are examples of secondary effects of this medication. The main drawbacks of MT are its high cost, the possibility of resistance because of its lengthy half-life (approximately one week) and the sustained presence of sub-therapeutic concentrations, and its teratogenicity.

Phospho lipid biosynthesis is impacted by MT's inhibition of phosphat idlylchioline biosynthesis. The first step in the suggested mechanism of action is binding to the cell membrane, which is followed by internalization via two membrane proteins: *L. donovani* The P4-ATPase subfamily includes the donovani miltefosine transporter (LdMT) and its putative noncatalytic β subunit (LdRos3). Both proteins are essential for the quick intracellular uptake of medications containing alkylphosphocholine, and they are mainly found in the plasma membrane of *Leishmania*. Phospholipids can more easily move from the exoplasmic to the cytoplasmic sites of the plasma membrane thanks to the stable protein complex formed by LdMT and LdRos3. It was also confirmed that MT inhibits mitochondrial cytochrome c oxidase, which lowers L's ATP levels and oxygen consumption rate.

Clinically resistant parasites have been reported in Nepal in cases of VL, even though MT has only recently entered the field. To predict the emergence of MT resistance and to describe the resulting mutants, in vitro resistance induction was previously carried out in the lab.

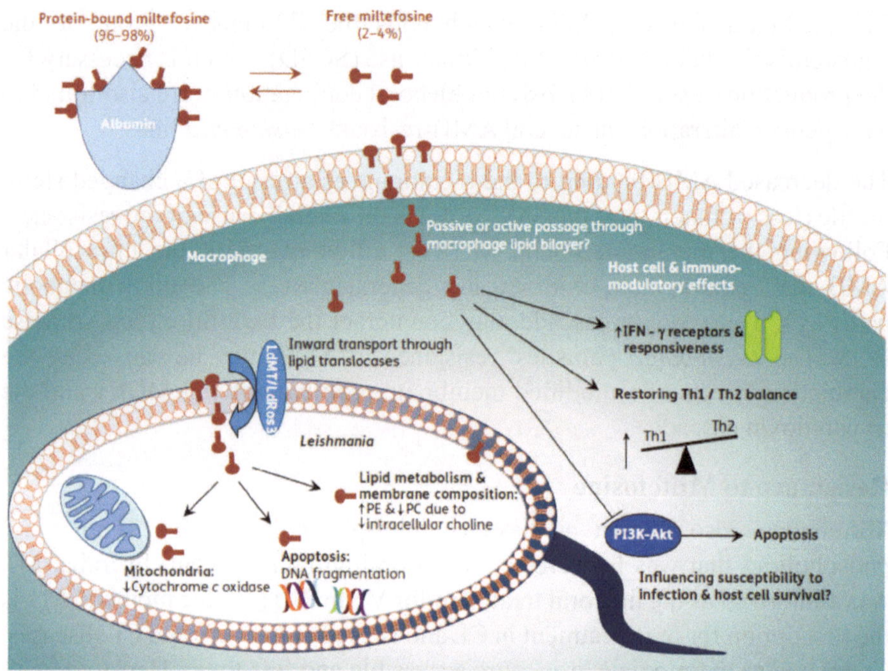


Antileishmanial mechanism of action of miltefosine. Source: Dorlo et al. (2012), J Antimicrob Chemother

### *Associated Mutations*

There have been reports of parasites from the Indian subcontinent that are less susceptible to MT. The confirmation of MT resistance in two cases of VL (*L. donovani*) in the lab enabled the isolates' phenotypic and genotypic characterization. Although there are very few MT-resistant clinical isolates, the strains' genomic and molecular profiles closely resemble those of laboratory-selected strains. Although the precise mechanism of MT resistance is unknown, all of the miltefosine-resistant *Leishmania* lines under investigation have shown evidence of decreased drug accumulation. This outcome could be the result of a different plasma membrane permeability, increased efflux, accelerated metabolism, or decreased drug absorption. A single point mutation in either of the two LdMT gene alleles is all that is needed to inactivate the transporter protein LdMT. The LdMT gene mutations L856P, T420N, and L832F showed an increased rate of resistance (both *in vivo* and *in vitro*), as well as changes in the lipid composition of the parasite membranes and decreased uptake, increased efflux, and faster metabolism. Additional mutations include Y354F and F1078Y in the LdMT gene, which were recently discovered, V176D, W210, and mutation M1 in LdRos3.

ABC transporter overexpression is one more mechanism linked to MT resistance. The *Leishmania* ABC transporters contain LMDR1/ABCB4, a P-glycoprotein-like transporter, which was the first molecule identified as being involved in experimental MT resistance. Increased resistance to MT in *Leishmania* is linked to overexpression of the ABC transporters ABCB4(MDR1), ABCG4, and ABCG6, which reduces intracellular accumulation by increasing drug efflux across the plasma membrane. Furthermore, changes in the sterol biosynthesis and membrane lipid composition in *MT-resistant L.* Drug-membrane interactions may also be impacted by Donovani promastigotes. Genes involved in phospholipid translocation and ergosterol biosynthesis have recently been proposed to contribute to resistance in *L. pneumoniae* through the use of cosmid-based functional cloning in conjunction with next-generation sequencing.

To get around the MT resistance, a number of compounds have been created. Sesquiterpenes have been shown to increase intracellular drug concentration by modulating new ABC transporteractivity, which can overcome multidrug resistance in *Leishmania*, including resistance to miltefosine. The over-expression of LMDR1 was demonstrated to be overcome by another flavonoid derivative at suboptimal dosages. By increasing intracellular drug accumulation, the 8-aminoquinoline sitamaquine overcomes LMDR1-mediated miltefosine resistance, demonstrating that sitamaquine is an effective reversal agent of LMDR1-mediated miltefosine resistance in *Leishmania* parasites.

## Resistance to Paromomycin

In 2006, the aminoglycoside antibiotic pomomycin (PMM) was introduced for the treatment of valamellar lung disease. In most cases, PMM is well tolerated, administered orally or intramuscularly, and rarely has side effects. Through its interactions with ribosomal subunits and promotion of ribosomal subunit association, PMM inhibits protein synthesis in bacterial infections. The binding to the major groove in the 16S rRNA in E's A-site was noticed. coli and the creation of mRNA misreading. But in the case of *Leishmania*, the mechanism of action is not entirely obvious. When PMM binds to the 16S ribosomal subunit in *Leishmania* parasites, it may inhibit protein synthesis by causing a local conformational change in the 16S ribosomal RNA's A site. The alterations at A1492 and A1493's N1 positions on the minor groove side of the A-site RNA suggested a translation-related mechanism of action. A number of additional mechanisms of action were suggested, including: a) altering the fluidity of membranes and lipid metabolism; b) lowering the potential of mitochondrial membranes; and c) respiratory dysfunction. The process of PMM uptake involves endocytosis and is aided by the binding of PMM to several parasite surface proteins, including prohibitin, paraflagellar rods (1D and 2D), and a P-type H+ATPase. The primary function of these proteins is to promote endocytosis and aid in the entry and retention of the drug within vacuoles.

Low cost, short administration time, good safety profile, and accessibility are some of the benefits that PMM offers. Nevertheless, paromomycin's physicochemical makeup hinders adequate concentration at the infection site. Utilizing solid lipid nanoparticles as a PMM delivery system has shown improved drug penetration into macrophages, boosted the immune response, and ultimately increased PMM effectiveness. In order to treat VL, a formulation comprising albumin microspheres loaded with PMM was created to target *Leishmania* parasites in macrophages. Compared to intramuscular injection, this formulation has the advantage of directly targeting macrophages, which reduces toxicity and causes less pain. Additionally, PMM was coupled to phosphatidylcholine (PC) liposomes that contained stearylamine (SA). PMM-SA-PM demonstrated no toxicity, superior antileishamanial activity, and an enhanced protective immunity effect.

### *Associated Mutations*

PMM resistance in prokaryotes has been linked to a number of processes, including enzymatic drug inactivation, ribosomal binding site mutations, and decreased drug accumulation. Although little is known about the resistance mechanisms in eukaryotic *Leishmania* parasites, it is believed that they involve a reduction in drug uptake. Numerous investigations revealed that PMN resistance in *L. donovani* is linked to a reduction in the drug's initial binding to the cell surface and a decrease in the drug's accumulation. Comparing resistant strains to PMM-sensitive strains, it was confirmed that there was an increase in the quantity of vesicular vacuoles and proteins involved in vesicular trafficking. High levels of glycolytic enzymes were also found, suggesting that the resistant strain gets its energy from either anaerobic or aerobic glycolysis. HSP70 family stress proteins were found to have higher basal levels in comparison to the sensitive strain. The most trustworthy theory of resistance contends that specific cell surface proteins are in charge of the drug's vacuole efflux after PMM is internalized through endocytosis. Consequently, a number of theories explain why *Leishmania* develops PMM resistance, including: a) translation rate modulation; b) interaction with vesicle-mediated trafficking; c) increased energetic metabolism via glycolysis; and d) effective protection provided by chaperone/stress-related proteins.

## Drug Targets & Innovative Approaches to Overcome Resistance

- The main treatment hazard for leishmaniasis has been identified as resistance to traditional therapeutic approaches. medication resistance may be overcome with the use of target-based medication delivery. If the following criteria can be met, the TSH system, polyamine production, surface lipids, and efflux pumps could all be made targets:
- The target must be crucial to the parasites' existence and survival;
- The target must be such that the mammalian host's complement is either nonexistent or sufficiently varied to allow for selective suppression;
- To improve the therapeutic efficacy of traditional therapeutic techniques, the target must overcome a credible resistance mechanism.

## Antitrypanosomal Drug Resistance

The tsetse fly is the vector for the neglected tropical disease known as human African trypanosomiasis (HAT), found in sub-Saharan Africa. There are two clinical variations of HAT: the slow-progressing form in West and Central Africa, which is brought on by *Trypanosoma brucei gambiense* (*T. b. gambiense*); and the more rapidly spreading form in Eastern and Southern Africa, which is brought on by *Trypanosoma brucei rhodesiense* (*T. b. rhodesiense*). The number of HAT cases increased since 1980s until 2006, when a notable decline was noted. WHO and numerous public and public-private organizations made excellent efforts for control, elimination, or eradication and the disease burden has decreased significantly in recent years. However, HAT is still a serious public health issue, if left untreated, can be fatal.

*T. brucei* cells have a single flagellum, a kinetoplast, a single mitochondrion with its own DNA, and a single central nucleus. This protozoan's life cycle alternates between an insect vector, the tsetse fly, and a mammal host. Tsetse flies can spread trypanosomes and are hemophagous in both sexes. When these flies consume trypanosomes found in the blood or skin of mammals, they contract the disease. Trypanosomes go through a number of intricate changes when they enter the fly's midgut and multiply before traveling to the salivary glands, which are home to the majority of the human-infective metacyclic forms. And when the fly bites a new human or animal host, the cycle is restarted.

HAT progresses through two main phases: An acute stage of the bloodstream and lymphatic system that affects the liver, spleen, and heart and is fatal to the host. The second stage of the disease, known as the "encephalitic stage", brought on by the trypanosomes capacity to penetrate the blood-brain barrier and reach the central nervous system. Meningoencephalitis is one of several neurological injuries seen at this stage. In the case of *T. b. rhodesiense*, this stage may appear in a few weeks however, in case of *T. b. gambiense* it may take a few months or several months to manifest. The virulence of the various *T. brucei* sub-species varies and causes a more severe and aggressive HAT and most likely death while *T. b. gambiense* takes longer to develop. It is unclear what motivation could account for the variations between the two. Highly immunogenic glycoproteins that cover the parasite cell membrane in the mammalian host have the ability to trigger a particular antibody response that destroys all parasites that are opsonized with these antibodies. Parasites have evolved an "antigenic-variation" to fend off this antibody-mediated immune response, wherein an antigenically distinct coat replaces the glycoprotein coat on the cell membrane. An irregular parasitemia, which manifests as irregular fevers, is the result of the interaction between the host's immune response and the parasite's antigenic variation.

The stage of the disease determines the kind of treatment. In the first stage of infection, it is preferable to administer safer medications; however, in the second stage, medications that can penetrate the blood-brain barrier and reach the parasite are needed. These medications are typically toxic and difficult to use. The disease may develop months after treatment because these protozoan may stay dormant in the host for an extended period of time and because of this, it is necessary to regularly analyse bodily fluids, including cerebrospinal fluid, and to monitor the patient for up to 24 months following treatment.

There are currently five medications used to treat HAT. For initial stage of *T. b. gambiense* and *T. b. rhodesiense* the medications that are advised are suramin and pentamidine. Eflornithine has been used as a monotherapy for the second stage of *T. b. gambiense* since 1990. As part of NECT (nifurtimox-eflornithine combination therapy), its use is currently recommended. NECT decreases treatment failure and eflornithine dosage, even though its effectiveness is comparable to that of eflornithine monotherapy. The only treatment for the second stage of *T. b. gambiense* and *T. b. rhodesiense* is melarsoprol, which has been in use since 1949 despite being extremely toxic and having cases of resistance documented in East Africa. The development of resistance to pentamidine and melarsoprol, which have been used for decades to treat African trypanosomiasis, is the primary reason for the urgent need for new medications despite the commendable efforts to control HAT. It is crucial to comprehend the mechanisms underlying resistance, especially cross-resistance.

Trypanosomes are incredibly versatile protozoa that have the remarkable capacity to adjust to drug pressure. Drug resistance may result from: (a) low drug levels within the cell (influx/efflux ratio); (b) changes to the drug's molecular target (linked to decreased activity); and (c) standard defence and repair systems. All medications used to treat trypanosomiasis, with the exception of eflornithine, have a multitarget effect, which lowers the rate of drug resistance development when compared to other infectious diseases. It is important to note that the zoonotic nature of the disease and the careless and inappropriate use of chemically similar medications in both humans and animals can be used to justify higher levels of drug resistance in rural and endemic areas.

### *Resistance to Pentamidine*

Pentamidine (PMD), which is also used to treat leishmaniasis, was initially developed to treat trypanosomiasis and is still used today. Despite some serious side effects patients tolerate it well. Pentamidine is more effective against *T. b. gambiense* (g-HAT) than *T. b. rhodesiense* (r-HAT) and has been used to treat the initial stage of HAT. Following internalization by endocytosis, PMD binds to the receptor aquaglyceroporin2 (AQP2) with affinity in the nM range, and a number of transporters, including the P2 adenosine/adenine, may aid in PMD uptake in trypanosomes. Active transport and endocytosis enable the intracellular build-up of PMD in DNA-containing compartments, such as the nucleus and the mitochondrion. As a DNA-binding medication, pentamidine causes the parasite mitochondrial membrane potential to collapse and induces the destruction of kinetoplast DNA.

### Associated Mutations

PMD uptake in species of *Trypanosoma brucei* is most likely caused by the P2 aminopurine transporter, and resistance to this agent has been linked to the transporter's malfunction. For the treatment of HAT, thepentamidine/ melarsoprol cross-resistance is a serious concern. Apart from the AT1/P2 transporter, AQP2, a surface protein primarily associated with osmoregulation, is also involved in pentamidine/melarsoprol cross-resistance.

### *Resistance to Suramin*

A polysulphonated symmetrical naphthalene derivative that is very useful in treating the initial stage of Trypanosomiasis is suramin. With the second-stage medications eflornithine, nifurtimox, and melarsoprol, suramin exhibits synergism. Suramin, on the other hand, prevents pentamidine from acting. The most likely target has been suggested to be glycolysis. On the other hand, the medication may target different pathways. For instance, the precise mechanism of action of suramin is unknown, but it is a competitive inhibitor of 6-phosphogluconated ehydrogenase, an enzyme of the pentose phosphate pathway. The lack of suramin resistance in humans may be explained by the theory that multiple enzymes are involved in the mechanism of action. Recently suramin was discovered to inhibit cytokinesis as *T. brucei* when exposed to the medication, shows cells with more than two nuclei, which suggested a cytokinesis defect with ongoing mitosis.

Aside from having a half-life of approximately 44–54 days and being in use for nearly a century, there have been no reports of suramin resistance in human pathogenic trypanosomes. In a lab setting, suramin-resistant strains were produced. It was confirmed that resistance may arise as a result of a variant surface glycoprotein (VSG) covering the blood stream form trypanosomes and shielding them from the immune responses of their mammalian hosts. The expression of the gene VSGSur was linked to suramin resistance following exposure to elevated suramin concentrations.

### *Resistance to Melarsoprol*

Inorganic arsenical compounds have been used for a long time; in 1858, they were first used to treat trypanosomiasis. Melarsoprol, also known as Mel B, was discovered in 1949 and is currently administered intravenously to treat rhodesiense and gambiense infections. Among its many unfavorable side effects, reactive encephalopathy is the most severe and potentially lethal. In West Africa, nifurtimox-eflornithine combination therapy (NECT) has largely replaced Mel B for the treatment of g-HAT due to the severe side effects, even though it is currently advised for the first stage of r-HAT and the second stage of g-HAT. The only proven treatment for advanced stage r-HAT in East Africa is still Mel B. NECT and Mel B are the only medications that can penetrate the blood-brain barrier and be used in the second stage of the disease; Mel B is the only medication that has demonstrated clinical resistance, especially in central Africa.

Mel B is a trivalent arsenical compound, and it's unclear exactly how it works. It has an affinity for sulfhydryl groups, particularly vicinal thiols found in proteins, but the effect is only mildly host- and parasite-specific in terms of cellular selectivity. The transporters P2 adenosine (AT1 gene) and aquaglyceroporin 2 (AQP2) of the parasite enable the selective uptake of MelB. Once inside the cell, it combines with trypanothione's dithiol group to form a complex that inhibits trypanothione redutase competitively. There isn't enough proof, though, to say that this process causes cell death. As an alternative, the parasite's glycolytic pathway may be connected to cell lysis. More recently, it was discovered that Mel B inhibited mitosis and that a particular set of kinases is required for this mitotic defect.

## Associated Mutations

The main mechanism of drug resistance in trypanosomes is loss of drug uptake. Defects in transporters P2 and AQP2 are accountable for the reduced uptake within the cell. Melarsoprolpentamidinecross resistance (MPXP) is present in HAT due to the fact that both medications share transporters, specifically AQP2. Mutations at the chimeric aquaglyceroporin AQP2-AQP3 and in the adenosine transporters P2 are linked to the resistance to Mel B.

### *Resistance to Eflornithine*

Eflornithine (also known as α-difluoromethylornithine, or DFMO) is the only treatment that is currently available for the second stage of Trypanosomiasis. *T. b. gambiense* HAT, when melarsoprol is not effective, it is used in conjunction with nifurtimox and is a significant advancement in terms of safer, more affordable, and simpler administration of medication. The mechanism of action of DFMO involves the selective and irreversible inhibition of ornithine decarboxylase (ODC), an enzyme involved in the regulation of proteins and nucleic acid synthesis, and necessary in the biosynthesis of the polyaminesspermidine and spermine. The sluggish turnover of ODC in *T. b. gambiense*, is the ability of DMFO to distinguish between human and parasite cells. Not surprisingly, *T. b. rhodesiense* does not seem susceptible to DFMO due to increased ODC turnover in this parasite. Unfortunately, DMFO's potential for developing clinical resistance is real if it is continued to be administered either by itself or in conjunction with nifurtimox.

### *Associated Mutations*

It was discovered that the transporters were essential for both drug sensitivity and resistance. In the lab, resistance to eflornithine was easily selected, suggesting a connection to amino acid transporters. The lack of the amino acid transporter TbAAT6 gene was discovered to be the cause of low DMFO uptake and sensitivity in resistant cases.

### *Resistance to Nifurtimox*

A nitrofuran known as nifurtimox, or Nfx, exhibits activity against African and American (i.e., *T. cruzi*), which causes Chagas disease, a form of trypanosomiasis. It appears that the effectiveness of nifurtimox for the chronic forms of the disease varies geographically, as better outcomes are seen in southern Brazil, Chile, Argentina, and Venezuela than in central Brazil. Nfx is exclusively registered for American trypanosomiasis, and its administration was only permitted in Africa upon national authorities' approval and acceptance of responsibility. However, since 2009, its use in conjunction with DMFO

(NECT) is advised for the treatment of g-HAT due to safety and efficacy data. NECT is made up of DMFO administered intravenously and Nfx administered orally.

As prodrugs, nitroheterocyclic compounds like Nfx need to be activated in order to exert their deadly effects. Although Nfx's exact mechanism of action is unknown, it may include reductive activation by bacterial-like nitroreductase (NTR) that is dependent on NADH and results in the creation of a cytotoxic, unsaturated open-chain nitrile derivative. The parasite may die as a result of oxidative damage brought on by free radicals produced by the one-electron reduction of the nitro group. It has recently been discovered that Nfx causes a significant disturbance of mitochondrial structure and function, which is consistent with damage to targets in the organelle where the drug is activated leading to a particular decrease in the amount of protein in the mitochondria.

**Associated Mutations**

A concentrated attempt was undertaken to clarify the possible mechanisms of Nfx medication resistance. Resistance is linked to a decrease in NTR activity, as demonstrated by laboratory-generated *T. cruzi* clones. Six genes were mostly found to be directly or indirectly related to the resistance mechanism to Nfx in *T. brucei*, with the NADH-dependent bacterial like nitroreductase (NTR) plays a major role in activating Nfx, which is linked to resistance.

***Resistance to Fexinidazole***

A 2-substituted 5-nitroimidazole known as fexinidazole (FEX) was discovered in the late 1970s to be a broad-spectrum anti-infective drug that also works against HAT. In preclinical tests, FEX shown strong effectiveness against *T. brucei*; nevertheless, it was discontinued because to its lack of economic feasibility. Nearly 30 years later, the Drugs for Neglected Diseases initiative (DNDi) screened a nitroheterocyclics library and found the same chemical again as a hit. The EMA's 2018 decision made it easier and supported the application for marketing authorization in endemic countries in 2019.

The sole oral medication that has been created and tested thus far to treat individuals with late-stage g-HAT is called FEX. Additionally, it is suitable for both the initial and subsequent stages of the illness. The simplicity of administration, which lessens the need for lumbar punctures, hospitalization, and other possible risks related to intravenous catheter use, may also have a favorable pharmacoeconomic effect. A Phase 3 evaluation of FEX for g-HAT is currently underway in Guinea and the Democratic Republic of the Congo.

Additionally, a study is being conducted in Spain to develop the medication for Chagas' illness. WHO is revising its treatment guidelines to clarify FEX's place in the present therapeutic arsenal.

Although FEX and its two metabolites, FEX sulfoxide and FEX sulfone, have been shown to limit DNA synthesis, their precise mode of action is uncertain. To exercise its selective activity against the parasite, FEX, like Nfx, needs to be bioactivated by NTR. A significant drawback of Nfx and FEX's method of action, which is based on the same NTR enzyme, is the potential for cross-resistance. The mechanisms of resistance to FEX were shown to be identical to those for Nfx in the laboratory.

## Strategies Available to Combat Drug Resistance

1) **Monitoring drug resistance**. Improved methods to monitor drug resistance that determine either the (i) phenotypic sensitivity of parasite isolates or (ii) molecular changes that indicate alterations in either the drug target or mechanisms that alter the intraparasite level of active drug are required.
2) **Monitoring therapy**
3) **Cost and distribution of drugs**
4) **Diagnostic methods**
5) **Combination therapies.** Drug combinations have proven to be an essential feature of antimicrobial treatment through design or use to (i) increase activity through use of compounds with synergistic or additive activity, (ii) prevent the emergence of drug resistance, (iii) lower required doses, reducing chances of toxic side effects and cost, or (iv) increase the spectrum of activity
6) New targets, new drugs. There are few better ways to avoid drug resistance than to have an adequate armory of drugs with different targets and no cross-resistance.

Global attempts to control and eradicate malaria are still seriously threatened by medication resistance. Recent findings show that, following an exceptional period of success in global malaria control, the decline of clinical cases has stalled, despite the fact that greater availability to effective malaria medicines has significantly contributed to the reduction of the malaria burden. Treatment failure for leishmaniasis is also becoming a bigger issue, made worse by the few available therapeutic alternatives, which are linked to toxicity, high cost, and developing drug resistance. The situation is similar in areas ravaged by trypanosomiasis, where current treatments are marked by severe toxicity and rising drug resistance linked, at least in part, to mutations that cause the transporters involved in drug import to lose their function.

For endemic nations, maintaining the effectiveness of the advised therapies for trypanosomiasis, leishmaniasis, and malaria is essential. The scientific community is nevertheless steadfast to stop the proliferation of parasites that are resistant to current medications. However, in order to achieve the ultimate goal of eradicating these parasite diseases, long-term measures are needed. In order to create safer and more alternative molecules, these tactics should involve a deeper comprehension of the mechanisms of action and resistance of clinical candidates and compounds that are already in more advanced phases of clinical trials. Furthermore, in order to expand the chemotherapeutic arsenal, get beyond safety restrictions, and combat the emergence of resistant parasites, novel compounds operating on hitherto unheard-of targets are desperately needed.

Perhaps the finest venues for sustaining R&D on novel drugs are public-private partnerships, which offer preclinical research knowledge and technical assistance for early-stage antibiotic drug discovery and product development. With any luck, these combined efforts will soon produce the intended results.

## Suggested Readings

Dorlo TP, Balasegaram M, Beijnen JH, de Vries PJ. (2012). Miltefosine: A review of its pharmacology and therapeutic efficacy in the treatment of leishmaniasis. J Antimicrob Chemother. 67(11):2576-97

Masoom Yasinzai, Momin Khan, Akhtar Nadhman and Gul Shahnaz (2013). Drug resistance in leishmaniasis: current drug-delivery systems and future perspectives.

Future Med. Chem. 5(15), 1877–1888

Rita Capela, Rui Moreira and Francisca Lopes (2019). An Overview of Drug Resistance in Protozoal Diseases. Int. J. Mol. Sci. 2019, 20, 5748

Tuvshintulga B, Sivakumar T, Yokoyama N, Igarashi I. (2019). Development of unstable resistance to diminazene aceturate in Babesia bovis. Int J Parasitol Drugs Drug Resist. 9:87-92

Velusamy R, Rani N, Ponnudurai G, Harikrishnan TJ, Anna T, Arunachalam K, Senthilvel K and Anbarasi P (2014). Influence of season, age and breed on prevalence of haemoprotozoan diseases in cattle of Tamil Nadu, India, VeterinaryWorld 7(8): 574-578.

# 8

# Role of Nutrition in Parasite Control

***Raju Kushwaha, Vinod Kumar, Muneendra Kumar, Shalini Vaswani, Avinash Kumar, Ram Dev Yadav and Mokshata Gupta***

*Department of Animal Nutrition, C.O.V.Sc. & A.H., DUVASU, Mathura Uttar Pradesh*

There are number of internal and external factors that affect the production performance of animals, among which parasites and parasitism are major of concern constraints to animal's productivity especially in tropical countries. Feed intake and nutrient requirements have been recognized for long time as an important parameter for determining the efficiency of animal production. Most of the parasitic infection in domestic animals is caused by gastro-intestinal nematode, which may result in depression in appetite, impairment in GI functions, alteration in protein, energy and mineral metabolism and changes in water balance. Nutrition can affect the ability of the host to cope with the consequences of parasitism and to contain and eventually to overcome parasitism. Since it is proposed that the host gives priority to the reversal of the pathophysiological consequences of parasitism over other body functions, it is to be expected that improved nutrition will always lead to improved resilience. On the other hand, it is proposed that the function of growth, pregnancy and lactation are prioritized over the expression of immunity. Improved nutrition may affect the degree of expression of immunity during these phases and can thus influence the resilience and resistance of host to parasite infection.

The role of nutrition in infectious diseases has been extensively investigated, as it is thought to affect establishment, pathogenesis, and duration of infections. The consensus is that under- or malnutrition impairs immunocompetence leading to increased susceptibility to and severity of infection. However, it becomes increasingly clear that disease patterns generated by the diet can be much more complex. Host-parasite interactions can be affected by the foraging activity per se, the amount of available food, as well as its quality. While the search for food often establishes the contact between host and pathogen, food quantity and quality may play a role later in the infection process. Infected hosts and their parasites compete for the same nutrients acquired by the host; i.e. nutrient supply could have direct effects on growth and reproduction of the host and simultaneously on the performance of the parasite. Moreover, certain components of the host's defence mechanisms could be affected by dietary nutrients and, in consequence, indirectly influence pathogen success. In contrast to what is often seen in mammals, food quantity limitation of the invertebrate host seems to impair the parasite, resulting in reduced within-host proliferation and decreased transmission. Although still in their early stage, the combined efforts of nutritional ecology and eco-immunological research have brought to light exciting aspects of food quality effects under parasite challenge in invertebrates.

### Host-parasite interactions

Host-parasite interactions are often seen as an open competition, with parasites attempting to overcome host resistance to infection. Herbivory is a common route of transmission of parasites that represents the most pervasive challenge to mammalian growth and reproduction. Many parasites have complex life cycles, i.e. they have to pass through several host species to reach maturity. Hence complex life cycles often consist of invertebrate and vertebrate hosts; the parasite likely varies in the machinery required for infection, exploitation and transmission of each host. The first difficulty for a parasite in a complex life cycle, compared to a single host system, is to successfully manage the additional transmission steps between hosts. Orally transmitted parasites often depend on predation of the current host by the next host. Therefore, to enhance transmission probability, parasites would profit from increased conspicuousness of the current host, at the time when the parasite is ready for transmission to the next host. After a parasite successfully found and orally entered the next host, an important step is the penetration of the intestinal mucosal wall. In each host, parasites have to survive the encounter with the host's immune system. If parasites with complex life cycles cope better with one of the different types of host immune systems, the parasite should perform differently in the other hosts. This substantiates the constraint of both hosts' immune systems on parasite performance and the impact on evolution of virulence in a parasite with a complex life cycle. There are great variations in life cycle, intermediary hosts, reproductive forms, and pathogenesis, which are responsible for differences in interaction between the host and the parasite, and the nature of the response of the host. The interaction between the host and nutrition can be broadly discussed from two interrelated perspectives, i) the effects of nutrition on the metabolic disturbances and pathophysiology induced by parasitism and ii) the influence of nutrient availability on the ability of the host to mount effective response against parasite establishment and/or development and to induce parasite rejection.

**a) Harmful effects of the parasite on the host**

Many parasites have harmful effects to their host, but in most cases these effects are not of such importance that the host is being killed. Such effects comprise:

i) Wasting disease: African trypanosomiasis and leishmaniasis may lead to severe loss of weight in both animals and man.

ii) Superinfections: In the case of cutaneous leishmaniasis ulcerations may lead to superinfections with bacteria

iii) Production of toxic compounds: It is thought that the African trypanosome, when in the central nervous system, produces aromatic amino-acid analogues that may influence brain function.

iv) Immunodepression: Malaria, bilharziosis, etc., lead to a certain degree of immune suppression which renders the infected host more susceptible to other diseases.

v) Allergic reactions: In the case of onchocerciasis (river blindness) the presence of the filarial worms under the skin may lead to depigmentation due to allergic reactions.

vi) Anaphylactic shock may be induced by the sudden release of large amounts of parasite internal antigens into the bloodstream.

vii) Also, drug treatment leading to a massive killing of the parasites may result in anaphylactic shock.

viii) Irritative reflexes (intestinal contractions: *Ascaris*)

ix) Irritation of skin and tissues by ecto and endoparasites and change the importance of the host for the community. Second, certain parasite species can be important in shaping parasite communities. Dominant parasite species can directly compete with other parasite species inside the host and reduce their abundance to some extent, and parasites that alter host phenotype can indirectly make the host more or less suitable for other parasite species. The possibility that a parasite species simultaneously affects the structure of all levels of the overall community, i.e. the parasite community and the community of free-living animals, is never considered. Given the many direct and indirect ways in which a parasite species can modulate the abundance of other species, it is conceivable that some parasite species have functionally important roles in a community, and that their removal would change the relative composition of the whole community.

**b) Beneficial effect of parasite to host**

Beside the harmful effects of parasite to host, many parasites are beneficial for host by different ways. First, it has been shown that parasites can have a role in structuring host communities. They can have differential effects on the different hosts that they exploit, they can directly debilitate a host that it is a key structuring force in the community, or they can indirectly alter the phenotype of their host and change the importance of the host for the community. Second, certain parasite species can be important in shaping parasite communities. Dominant parasite species can directly compete with other parasite species inside the host and reduce their abundance to some extent, and parasites that alter host phenotype can indirectly make the host more or less suitable for other parasite species. The possibility that a parasite species simultaneously affects the structure of all levels of the overall community, i.e. the parasite community and the community of free-living animals, is never considered. Given the many direct and indirect ways in which a parasite species can modulate the abundance of other species, it is conceivable that some parasite species have functionally important roles in a community, and that their removal would change the relative composition of the whole community.

## Malnutrition and Parasitic Infections

Malnutrition and parasitic infections are directly related. Malnutrition occurs in cases of gastro-intestinal (GI) parasitic infections due to induction of intestinal bleeding, impaired digestion and poor absorption of nutrients. These parasites also lead to reduction in feed intake, fat absorption, protein usage and loss of nutrients in the form of diarrhoea. Likewise, malnutrition adversely affects local and systemic immune responses, resulting in increased susceptibility to parasitic infections. GI parasites are one of the major risk factors which contribute to malnutrition, reduced performance and poor productivity in livestock and poultry. In human populations, malnourished people are primarily at risk of getting heavy parasitic infections, and helminthic infections with *Ascaris lumbricoides*, hookworms, *Trichuris trichiura* and *Schistosoma mansoni* usually cause malnutrition in humans.

Among environmental factors, nutritional status plays an important role in affecting resistance to infection. Protein malnutrition in this regard is of prime consideration, as it leads to poor immunity and increased parasite burden.

The public and veterinary health significance of helminth infections are often studied in the laboratory with the model roundworm, *Heligmosomoides polygyrus* in mice. This parasitic infection may result in poor growth. The parasite load varies in different strains of the mice, representing genetic variation for resistance.

## Nutritional Status and the Host-Parasite Relationship

The study of pathogenic trypanosomes of man and animals, and the search for effective chemotherapeutic agents, has commanded the attention of investigators during recent years. The studies on carbohydrate metabolism and respiration have been done on pathogenic and non-pathogenic trypansomes produced by animal infections and by culture, and several studies have dealt with the physiology of the host during infection. Comparative studies on the oxygen consumption and carbohydrate metabolism of trypanosome species have revealed a considerable range of activity. The non-pathogen, *T. lewisi,* has a low glucose consumption and a high respiratory quotient. The pathogen, *T. rhodesiense* (blood stream form), consumes glucose rapidly (range 1.0-1.5 mg. per 100 million per hour), but the respiratory quotient is 0.16. The high carbohydrate utilization and end products produced by the pathogenic species are shedding some light on the mechanisms of pathogenicity. *T. cruzi* and the non-pathogen *T. lewisi* converted glucose into lactic, acetic, and succinic acids, and the intermediate species, *T. congolense* and *T. vivax* (animal pathogens) produce glycerol, acetic acid, and succinic or lactic and pyruvic acids.

In a study on the catabolism of glucose by four strains of *T. rhodiesense*, these investigators showed conclusively that pyruvate is the main end product of glucose metabolism in vivo. Abnormally high blood pyruvate levels could be correlated with the intensity of infection. Since the levels returned to normal after treatment with a specific drug, the conclusion was reached that, the pyruvate produced by the parasite is greater than the amount that the host can metabolize or excrete. This result is suggestive of a mechanism of pathogenesis by this organism for its host. When evidence becomes available about the protein and nucleic acid metabolism and the end products formed, a more intelligent approach will be possible to experimentation to explain the morbidity and mortality of African sleeping sickness. Since one of the frustrating characteristics of trypanosomes is their ability to develop resistance to chemotherapeutic agents, it might equally be true that they are highly adaptive in their metabolic pathways and consequently their end products and disease-producing capacity will be equally different. Although the reactions of the resistant strain to enzyme inhibitors were essentially unchanged, this strain of parasite showed a slight increase in sensitivity to cyanide and a definite increase in sensitivity to two nitrofurans. Another difficulty in studying experimental trypanosomiasis has been the difficulty in reproducing central nervous system lesions and symptoms. The blood stream infections are believed to be too short for the development of the characteristic lesions seen in the human disease. Thus, a way has been found to compare chemotherapeutic, biochemical, and pathological results of infection by *T. gambiense* in the same host.

## Consequences of Nutrition on the Parasite Environment

Parasites identify and select precise locations to reside within their hosts. Although the exact reasons for the specific choice of habitat are still not clear, the specificity of the location is so consistent that cannot be disputed. Consequently, we may assume that any changes in the environment of the parasites may affect the incoming or the resident parasite population in two ways. The first one is by influencing the ability of incoming parasites to identify their niche thereby inhibiting their abilities to feed and reproduce. The second one is by creating a hostile/toxic environment for the incoming or resident parasites, with detrimental consequences on their survival. For example, changes in the levels or types of sugars in the diets of parasitized rats resulted in parasites changing location in the gut and consequentially experiencing penalties in their growth and reproduction. Unfortunately, this research did not explore the mechanisms that underlined these observations or the manner in which the specific carbohydrates affected the environment of the parasites. The specific conditions that carbohydrates create in the gastrointestinal tract of parasitised hosts attracted attention, the changes in fermentation patterns in the large intestine of pigs altered pH in various compartments of the gastrointestinal tract and reduced parasite populations. They showed that the consumption of diets high in inulin, a highly degradable fructose polymer, reduced worm numbers and egg counts in pigs infected with the large intestine nematode *Trichuris suis*. Similarly, infusion of short chain fatty acids (SCFA) and lactate acid (LA), which are the fermentation products of inulin, also reduced populations of Oesophagostomum dentatum in pigs. The specific mode of action of the fermentation products in regulating the parasites is not clear. It was proposed that SCFA and LA may exert some direct effects on worm physiology, especially the females. High inulin diets were detrimental to parasites during the establishment of an infection and on patent infections. In addition, following the consumption of inulin and the infusion of the SCFA and LA, pH was reduced in the caecum and the proximal colon of the pig. The close association between increased levels of SCFA and LA, low pH and expulsion of nematodes suggests that changes in pH may play a major role in worm expulsion, perhaps by creating an unsuitable environment for mature and immature parasites.

As with carbohydrate fermentation in monogastrics, changes in rumen pH may affect parasite establishment or survival. For example, the ekdysis of infective larvae, otherwise known as exsheathment, is a process necessary for the successful establishment in the host. Exsheathment generally occurs in the rumen for many of the gastrointestinal nematodes of small ruminants, including *Haemonchus contortus*, *Teladorsagia* spp. and *Trichostrongylus* spp. Changes in pH of the rumen, as well as bicarbonate concentrations, influence this process. In addition, dietary changes affect the exsheathment kinetics of gastrointestinal nematodes in ruminants. Dietary changes associated with changes in rumen pH, such as excessive carbohydrate ingestion, should be further considered for their antiparasitic potential. However, this should be done in combination with their antinutritional effects, modulated via negative consequences to rumen microflora, prior to advocating them as potential means for parasite control.

In addition to carbohydrate consumption, dietary protein may influence conditions in the gastrointestinal tract thereby affecting parasite survival in ruminants. This effect of protein would be in addition to the well-established role of protein in resistance and resilience. The protein supplementation reduced the level of parasitism in lambs and also that high-protein diets increased production of ammonia in rumen digesta. They suggest accumulated ammonia in the rumen might directly influence the rumen microenvironment by exhibiting toxic effects on *Haemonchus contortus*. High rumen ammonia also increases the pH of the rumen, which may also affect the exsheathment of the infective larvae as discussed earlier. In addition to protein excess, extreme protein deficiency may create an unfavorable environment for parasites. The very low protein content of the food may have altered the structure and/or the physiology of the gut and may have created an unsuitable and hostile environment for the survival of parasites. Low-protein diets may change the morphology of the gastrointestinal mucosa, influence local blood flow and increase epithelial cell apoptosis, all of which may affect parasite establishment and survival. However, as none of the above hypotheses were further investigated to elucidate the possible mechanisms, it is not possible to reject or accept them. Consequently, there may be more to the role of protein in parasite regulation than the effects on resilience and resistance, and future efforts should explore the full potential of protein nutrition in parasite control.

### a) Influence of Nutrition on Parasite Establishment

The nature of the immune response to gastrointestinal nematodes varies considerably at different stages of infection. The stages include effectors against parasite establishment, effectors against existing mature infections and effectors against reinfection. There is evidence to suggest that the influence of nutrition varies with these different stages. To date, much of this evidence has been obtained from experimental studies in housed animals where the diet and level and type of infection can be controlled. This section considers the effects of diet on parasite establishment in naive animals. This can be determined most easily in studies in which a single infection is given to animals which have already been established on specific diets. In other situations, in which trickle (continuous or repeated) infections are given it is more difficult to distinguish between the effects on initial infection and the responses to mature and new infections, although it is recognised that trickle infections more closely resemble the situation in the field. The general consensus from these various studies is that protein intake does not appear to influence initial parasite establishment in ruminant, although the pathophysiological consequences are usually more severe in animals on lower planes of protein intake.

**b) Influence of Nutrition on Established Infections**

An observation was that chronic haemonchosis was associated with reduced feed quality during the dry season suggested that changes in nutrient intake could influence established infections. This observation has been repeated in other tropical areas where a fall in feed quality during the dry season is frequently associated with severe parasitism despite low or negligible larval intake. The basis of these observations has not been examined under experimental conditions but may result from dietary-induced immunosuppression which prevents the elimination of established infections. Early evidence that a high level of dietary protein may be beneficial to animals with established infections was provided by investigations into the influence of diet on the recovery of housed sheep with heavy mixed infections which were acquired whilst at grass. In all the studies reported to date in which experimental trickle (continuous)-infections have been given over prolonged periods the plane of nutrition has been established prior to infection and maintained unchanged throughout the study, so it has not been possible to evaluate accurately the influence of nutrition on established infections. However, in such studies there is evidence that the level of dietary protein intake significantly affects the immune response and this is reflected in reduced faecal egg counts, reduced worm burdens and enhanced resistance to reinfection in animals receiving diets with higher levels of protein. We believe there is a need to examine, under controlled experimental conditions, the impact that changes in nutrient intake may have on established infections since seasonal changes in feed quality and quantity are likely to have significant influences on the responses of the host to its parasite burden and the epidemiology of the infection.

### c) Effect of Nutrition on Host Resilience

Maintenance of body protein is expected to have the highest priority for nutrient allocation because it guarantees animal survival in the short term. Growth and reproduction are given the second highest priority because they ensure the preservation of the animal's genetic material in the long term. Functions regulating the parasite population (expression of immunity) will be greatly influenced by host nutrition, because they are expected to be given a lower priority for a scarce resource allocation than the functions of maintenance, growth or reproduction. This framework proposes that the provision of additional nutrients would lead to improved resilience. Evidence from both indoor and grazing trials on sheep additional dietary protein supports this concept. In ruminant hosts, dietary nitrogen is either degraded in the rumen and used by microorganisms or is passed undegraded (bypass protein). Microbial and bypass protein form sources of metabolizable protein for absorption in the small intestine. Housed sheep experimentally infected with a single or 'trickle' dose of larvae of either abomasal (i.e. in the abomasum, the fourth ruminant stomach) or intestinal nematodes showed less-severe pathophysiological consequences of infection when the supply of metabolizable protein to the intestine was increased by feeding undegradable protein. Reductions in blood parameters such as haematocrit, total serum protein and albumin concentrations were less marked in animals offered a high level of metabolizable protein than in animals on low to moderate protein rations. Production responses such as live-weight gain, wool growth and carcass quality have also been improved by protein supplementation of either housed animals infected daily with a 'trickle' nematode infection or in naturally infected grazing livestock. Positive effects of protein supplementation on resilience to nematode infection have also been recorded in goats. Similar improvements in resilience of parasitized sheep have resulted from the supplementation of a basal diet with urea, a source of degradable nitrogen. Although these responses to urea supplementation were less than those obtained with high-quality undegradable proteins, this approach is feasible in many tropical and subtropical areas where poor quality forages are generally available and the cost of high-quality protein supplements is prohibitive.

Experiments show that, in general, the improvements in resilience caused by dietary supplementation with protein are greatest in young, naive animals, in which pathophysiological disturbances to the GI tract such as protein-losing gastroenteritis and changes in gut function are most pronounced. There is also indirect evidence of improved resilience in breeding ewes supplemented with protein. There is compelling evidence that dietary protein, is more important than energy in improving resilience, although, if the animal is severely undernourished, increasing energy supply will obviously have an effect on resilience. In this context, it is of interest that growing sheep experimentally infected with *Trichostrongylus colubriformis* could alter their diet selection from two isoenergetic foods differing in their protein content. The parasitized sheep selected a higher proportion of a high protein food in their diet than did uninfected controls, thus enabling them to improve their resilience to infection. It has been suggested that increases in protein intake have not always influenced the resilience of livestock to parasitic infection. In some cases, the calculated difference in metabolizable protein supply between supplemented and unsupplemented animals was too small to warrant a major effect and, in others, insufficient nutritional information is provided to make a valid judgement. We conclude that, in cases of protein scarcity, supplementation with additional (metabolizable) protein will indeed lead to improvement of resilience of parasitized animals.

**d) Effect of Nutrition on Host Resistance**

Hosts invariably develop some resistance to a parasite following continuous exposure and this will be influenced by the age, breed and productive state of the animal. A number of studies have addressed the relationship between the nutritional status of the host and its ability to regulate a parasite infection. The nutrient partioning framework considered earlier helps to explain the results from the literature in terms of the different requirements of the host, particularly for protein, during different phases of its life cycle. Although the acquisition and expression of immunity is a continuum, it is useful to separate the possible nutrient requirements associated with initial responses to parasite invasion in a naive animal from those that occur during expression or maintenance of resistance in hosts who have acquired immunity.

**e) Influence of Nutrition on Immune Responses to Parasites**

It is well established that the nutritional status of the host can influence the rate of acquisition of immunity to parasitic and other infections in man and many animal species and that dietary protein is of particular importance. It seems reasonable to suggest that there may be competition for available nutrients between the requirement to mount an effective immune response and the maintenance of growth in the young parasitised animal which has a high metabolizable protein requirement relative to energy demand. Once the animal's rate of growth declines and it starts to attain a mature body weight, the demands of the immune response may be able to be more fully satisfied. This partitioning of available nutrients between growth and immune responses could in part explain the immune unresponsiveness of the young ruminant to gastrointestinal nematode infection. The addition of a "protected" protein would increase the availability of amino acids at the small intestine and possibly enable the young growing lamb to mount a more effective immune response. The acquisition of immunity will have a cost penalty but currently we have no quantitative estimates of this penalty where animals are maintaining their immune competence under continuous larval challenge.

### f) Influence of Nutrition on Expression of Genotype

Even when maintained on similar planes of nutrition ruminants show considerable variation in susceptibility to parasitic infections as a result of genetic variation. With the increasing interest in the exploitation of genetically resistant livestock to control helminthosis and the findings that low planes of nutrition can exacerbate the pathogenic effects of gastrointestinal helminthosis it is important to determine if the benefits of genetic resistance are easily lost when nutrition is sub-optimal. The results clearly show that protein supplemented diets can significantly reduce the pathophysiological changes associated with haemonchosis in genetically susceptible and genetically resistant animals. However, these effects are more pronounced in the former breeds and less critical in the latter breeds. This indicates that the benefits of a superior genotype are not lost on a low protein diet whilst a high protein diet can help overcome the disadvantages of an inferior genotype.

## Nutritional strategy to Control Parasitism

### a) Nutrient-partitioning Framework

Effects of microbial protein (MP) supply on resistance to gastrointestinal nematodes can be viewed within a nutrient-partitioning framework, which introduces the concept of prioritization for the allocation of scarce resources toward different bodily functions; the higher the priority, the less likely host nutrition would affect the bodily function. Animals would be expected to give the highest priority to the allocation of scarce resources for maintenance functions, i.e. maintenance of body protein, as this will guarantee survival in the short term. This would include the repair and/or replacement of damaged and/or lost host tissue caused by parasitic infestation. Traditionally, immune functions have been regarded as part of the collectively termed "maintenance functions", and hence would be expected to be prioritized over other bodily functions. However, since at least some aspects of immunity are sensitive to changes in MP supply, immune functions are in this framework considered separately from maintenance. Thus, once scarce nutrient allocation to maintenance has been fulfilled, the remaining scarce resources would need to be allocated to bodily functions associated with growth, reproduction and immunity to parasites. The growing animal that encounters parasites for the first time would be expected to prioritize scarce resource allocation to the acquisition of immunity over growth; otherwise, it may succumb to the adverse consequences of parasitism before reaching reproductive maturity. However, once immunity has been acquired, growth and reproduction would be prioritized over expression of immunity to parasites, as the former bodily functions ensure preservation of the host's genetic material. This framework puts forward various hypotheses on the effects of MP nutrition on resistance to gastrointestinal nematodes. The difference between priority for scarce resource allocation to acquisition and expression of immunity relative to productive functions, leads to the hypothesis that changes in MP supply would not be expected to affect the rate of acquisition of immunity, but would greatly affect expression of immunity to gastrointestinal nematodes. Also, it can be hypothesized that expression of immunity will be penalized at times of increased nutrient requirements of the prioritized reproductive effort. The latter implies that the periparturient breakdown of immunity to gastrointestinal nematodes, which results in increased worm burdens and nematode egg excretion around parturition, may have a nutritional basis.

### b) Enhancing feed and Nutrient Intake

Adequate plane of nutrition is one of very basic aspect which modulates the nutritional status and health of the animals. The animals gradually recover with the gradual increase in feed intake and body weight. The animals ultimately become apparently normal due to their normal immunocompetence mechanism. Therefore, there should be selection of feed ingredients that are palatable or supplementation of appetite enhancer (molasses, micronutrients, processed feed ingredients, flavours, colours etc.) to restore in parasitized animals and also provision of concentrated nutrients (energy and protein) in the feed consumed by the animals to meet the minimum maintenance need during a disease process.

### c) Protein Supplementation and Parasitism

The suggestion that acquisition, but not expression, of immunity takes priority over growth implies that changes in MP supply, would be expected to affect faecal eggs counts (FEC) and worm burdens only during the phase of expression of immunity. Thus, effects of MP supply on the level of gastrointestinal nematode parasitism would be expected to show temporal effects; an increased MP supply would reduce FEC and worm burdens only at later stages in experimental parasitic infestations. Casein infused in the abomasum of growing *Trichostrongylus colubriformis* infested sheep for 12 weeks reduced worm burdens by 55% at week 12, but worm burdens were not affected at week 6. Fishmeal supplementation to *T. colubriformis* infested sheep resulted in 44 and 99% reduced worm burdens at weeks 15 and 20, respectively, but worm burdens did not differ at weeks 5 and 10. Indeed, increasing dietary MP supply to *Teladorsagia circumcincta* infested, lactating ewes, from 0.65 to 1.25 times their assumed MP requirements, resulted in increased milk production for the first MP increments only, whilst only the last increment resulted in a reduced worm burden. Unlike in growing lambs, there is only limited evidence in support of the view that protein supplementation affects immune effector responses in periparturient ewes, although the limited evidence available suggest that protein supply results in increased numbers of globule leukocytes. The aforementioned outcomes have been observed through supplementation with a wide range of protein sources, including soybean meal, fishmeal, cottonseed meal and urea. The magnitude of these effects would be dependent on the degree of MP scarcity. As such, it would be expected that the largest benefit from protein supplementation would be expected in multiple-rearing ewes in a relatively poor body condition and in growing lambs with a high potential for growth.

### d) Nutritional Enhancement of Immunity to Parasitism

Modulating immunity of the animal to the infection by nutritional manipulation is one of the latest modus operandi in control and prevention of parasitism disease. Acquired immunity in the host has effects on parasite establishment, development, survival and fecundity. The duration of the phase of acquisition of immunity, during which the immune system recognizes the parasite and the changes that precede an effective immunological response could vary greatly from a few days in protozoan infection to several weeks in helminth infection. Nutrition of the host could have the potential to affect how rapidly immunity is acquired and expressed in defense of the parasitism. Under normal nutritional circumstances, changes in nutrient intake would not be expected to affect the early rate of acquisition of immunity to parasites in young animals. However, in severely undernourished animals that loose protein mass, the acquisition of immunity is severely impaired. There is a large inter-animal variation in the rate of development of resistance both within the same breed and between breeds which appear to have a strong genetic basis. Host protein and energy nutrition can affect greatly, the expression of immunity in cattle, sheep. The supplementation of a hay diet with 150 g protected protein or 100 g fish meal per day affected the rate of worm expulsion after 10 weeks of trickle infection with *T. colubriformis* and the apparent rate of expulsion was related to the level of supplementation. As many components of the effecter arm of the immune system such as immunoglobulins, mucoproteins and cellular products (leukotrienes) are all proteinaceous moieties, they would be expected to draw on protein resources both in quantitative and qualitative terms. Immune system has also some specific requirements for certain micronutrients such as Zn, Fe, Se.

### e) Supplementing Micronutrients

Supplementation of minerals and vitamins can play a key role in affecting ruminant susceptibility. Studies on the relationship of phosphorous (P) with *T. vitrinus* worm burden in sheep suggest that increased P supply decreases mean worm burden. Trace elements (TEs) like Cu, Mo, and Se are known to influence the host resistance to nematode infection with a probable direct anthelmintic effect and by influencing host metabolism. The worm burden reduced (*H. contortus, O. circumcincta*) in lambs by administering copper oxide wire particles in the diet. The worm burden of *H. contortus* reduced and *T. colubriformis* in browsing goats supplemented with copper oxide needles. In caecal coccidiosis (*E. tenella*), an increased levels of selenium and vitamin E found to reduce the severity of primary infection and improve weight gain and feed conversion. Vitamins A, D, and B complex are integral in developing immunity to parasites. Essential minerals include cobalt, used to synthesize vitamin B12, and iron. It is also observed that when the phosphorus level of the diet was at a level of 0.28% phosphorus on a dry matter basis, the weight gain of lambs infected with parasites was increased by 40% over those lambs fed a low (0.18%) phosphorus level diet.

In the abomasum, parasites present in the growing stages can affect P and Ca absorption, resulting in skeletal defects. Sheep infected with larvae of *Ostertagia circumcincta* showed a deficiency of Ca and P, but in the case of *Trichostrongylus colubriformis* infected sheep, along with Ca and P deficiency, inhibition of skeletal development was also recorded. Low levels of Co, Zn, and Fe in sheep infected with Fasciolosis have been observed. Rams infected with *H. contortus* showed a significant effect on the mean levels of Zn, Co, Se and Cu. It has been stated that TEs may be used for effective and quick cure against GI parasitic infection. Administration of Cu, Se and vitamin E in sheep showed a significant increase in immunity against *H. contortus*. For the physiological functioning of the immune system, several micro and macro TEs are required. Essential TEs are important for cell metabolism and the immune system. Adequate levels of TEs, such as selenium, molybdenum, copper, iron, zinc and cobalt have significant effects on animal health through reduced GI parasitic infection. Other TEs are either directly or indirectly involved via physiological pathways that regulate mucosal immunity. The likelihood that minerals can affect gut immune responses of livestock against endoparasites can be predicted through implications generated in epidemiological and experimental studies in ruminants and monogastric species. Understanding immunity and nutrition is necessary for prevention of diseases.

It has been reported that deficiency of TEs in animals is directly associated with depressed immune system. Nutrition has the potential to affect GI parasites because it directly affects the degree of expression of the immunity and rate of acquisition of the infection, which can reduce the survival, fecundity, and establishment of GI parasites. A gap between TE deficiencies and parasitic infections in animals is reviewed in this chapter, which confirms the requirement for further research to explain their possible role against GI parasites. Due to sub-clinical deficiencies of TEs, animals use feed less efficiently, which may lead to a decrease in growth rate, low reproductive performance, and immunodeficiency. However, acute deficiencies of TEs cause huge economic losses in the sense of mortality. Therefore, it is important to identify TE-enriched pasture and soil to improve the immunity in animals. Animals having inadequate supplies of nutrients are more prone to GI parasitic infections, which reduce their productivity. To determine the sufficient amount of TEs for animals, appropriate analyses of soil, forages, and animals are essential. Nutrition of animals depends upon soil-plant-animal complex, although season can strongly influence the dietary requirements for TEs. Deficiencies of TEs in soil and forages affect animal production adversely. Analysis of a particular area is imperative to assess its TE profile and to compare their availability for grazing animals.

### f) Use of Herbal Feed Additives

Herbs have been used for years by farmers and traditional healers to treat parasitism and improve performance of livestock, and many modern commercial medicines are derived from plants. However, scientific evidence on the antiparasitic efficacy of most plant products is limited, regardless of their wide ethnoveterinary usage. The possible positive effects of plant secondary metabolites (PSM) as additives in the livestock rationing include antioxidant and anthelminthic properties and complex formation between protein and condensed tannins that protects dietary protein from degradation by the symbiotic microflora of foregut fermenters, increasing its utilisation by the animal. This protein effect is probably only beneficial to animals under a narrow range of nutrient-rich conditions found mainly in agricultural systems. *In vivo* controlled studies have shown that plant remedies have in most instances resulted in reductions in the level of parasitism much lower than those observed with anthelmintic drugs. Although in many cases the active compounds in the herbal remedies have not been fully identified, plant enzymes, such as cysteine proteinases, or secondary metabolites, such as alkaloids, glycosides and tannins have shown dose-dependent anti-parasitic properties. However, as some of the active compounds may also have anti-nutritional effects, such as reduced food intake and performance, it is essential to validate the anti-parasitic effects of plant products in relation to their potential anti-nutritional and other side effects. Condensed tannins (CT) have shown biological effects that may aid in the control of dewormer-resistant internal parasites (IP) and thus CT in forages have potential to be a component of IP control programs. Plant CT may have direct or indirect effects on IP. Direct effects might be mediated through CT-nematode interactions affecting physiological functioning of IP. *In-vitro* and *in-vivo* studies have shown that CT in several temperate and tropical forages can inhibit infective gut worm larvae of sheep and goats and both gut and lung worms in farmed deer, with effects influenced by both concentration and structure of CT. It is suggested that Calliandra could reduce faecal egg counts of lambs infected with *T. colubriformis*, and that such an effect is mediated probably by some direct toxic or physiological effect of the legume rather than by improvement in protein nutrition. Indirectly, CT can improve protein nutrition by binding to plant proteins in the rumen and preventing microbial degradation, thereby increasing amino acid flow to the duodenum.

Several ovine studies have shown that improved protein nutrition reduces parasite infestation. This is assumed to be mediated by enhanced host immunity, which may be especially important with selection for immunity to IP. Saponin mixtures present in plants and plant products like Fenugreek, Sesbania, Soapnut etc. possess diverse biological effects and it is observed to be detrimental to protozoa. This property could be exploited in treatment of protozoal infections in other animals. Triterpenoid and steroid saponins have been found to be detrimental to several infectious protozoans such as *Plasmodium falciparum, Giardia* trophozoites and *Leishmania* species. The toxicity of saponins to protozoans seems to be widespread and non-specific and is obviously the result of their detergent effect on the cell membranes. A mixture of essential oils from clove (1.0%), thyme (0.1%), peppermint (0.1%) and lemon (0.1%) observed to have effects on coccidia oocyte output and the number of *Clostridium perfringens* in broiler chicks when artificially inoculated. A lot of other bioactive components, viz. terpenes, triterpenoides, alkaloids, etc. has variable effects as antimicrobial agents. The possible antiparasitic role of these compounds cannot be ruled out. It has also been said that there may be a synergistic effect of two or more components against intestinal parasitism.

## Effect of Parasitism on Host

### a) Effect on Feed Intake

Feed intake of *Trypanosoma vivax* infected sheep was depressed at both plane of nutrition i.e. 12% for males, and 17% and 22% for (pregnant and lactating) females. It was observed that an average feed intake per unit metabolic body size reduced by 13 to 24% in goat 2 weeks after infection with *T. vivax*. About 20 % reduction in feed intake during febrile trypanosomiasis was recorded in goats and in sheep. A difference was observed in food intakes between *T. vivax* infected and control groups in the last week before parturition, with 22% and 19% lower than control groups. Factors responsible for a reduced feed intake during trypanosomiasis are not known but it may be due to cachectin or TNF, bradykinin, fever and stress produced by the host and toxin released by the *T. brucei*.

### b) Effect on Nutrient Utilization

Gastro-intestinal parasitism affects the nutrient utilization of host in many ways, viz.

i) Reduce nutrient availability to the host through reduction in voluntary feed intake and/ or reduction in the efficiency of absorbed nutrients.

ii) Increased loss of endogenous protein into the GI tract, partly as a result of leakage of plasma protein, and partly due to increased mucoprotein production and sloughing of epithelial cells in to the alimentary tract.

iii) Effect on GI motility causing diarrhoea enhances the loss of plasma protein, sodium and chloride with increase in potassium level thereby altering acid-base balance.

iv) An increase in metabolic protein/ amino acids requirement as a consequence to endogenous protein loss and

v) Diversion of nutrients and protein synthesis from production processes such as muscle, bone, wool, milk, egg, etc. towards repairment/ replenishment of local tissue injury at GI level, mucus secretion and/ or loss of plasma or blood and other defensive and immunomodulatory system during parasitism.

### c) Effect on Energy Metabolism

The major metabolic consequence of parasitism, especially of the blood-borne parasites is an increase in energy (maintenance) requirements due to increase in heat increment as a result of fever. A 15% rise in metabolic rate and 25% rise in maintenance requirement for every degree rise in body temperature have been reported. Reductions in the digestion of the gross energy of the complete diet have been frequently reported in a range of helminths infections in both cattle and sheep. The gross efficiency of utilization of ME for growth was reduced by 30 and 37 % for *O. circumcincta* and *T. colubriformis* infections respectively. Increased heat production may be expected to accompany the increases in protein turnover, but there appear to be no reports of such increases. A detailed investigation of the partitioning of dietary energy in subclinical haemonchosis using direct calorimetry showed faecal and urinary energy losses not to be significantly reduced by infection with *H. contortus* /kg live weight, nor was there any effect on heat production. However, infected animals lost a greater proportion of dietary energy as methane. Energy retention and the efficiency of utilization of ME for gain purposes were not significantly different. Unfortunately, the establishment of the infection was particularly low in this study. Level of feed intake affects heat production and where the gross efficiency of energy utilization was apparently impaired in infected animals this was largely because of reduced intake. However, net efficiency of utilization of ME for production (i.e. feed ME less maintenance cost) is related to the energy density of the complete diet, and in the calorimetry, findings reviewed derived maintenance and net efficiency values were extremely varied and generally not related to infection. Findings from carcass evaluation however, show infected animals to have lower energy retention. There is clearly a shortage of information and understanding of energy metabolism in parasitized ruminants.

It was observed that adequate dietary energy ameliorates the disease produced by *T. brucei* in growing pigs as during 8-week post infection. Lipids constitute 15-20% of trypanpsomal dry weight. They obtain cholesterol from the host by uptake and degradation of low density or high-density lipoproteins. Trypanosome requires cholesterol for growth and multiplication and is the main sterol in trypanosomes identified a Phospholipase- A1 in *T. cruzi* and they observed that its concentration is high in pathogenic trypomastigote and amastigote trypanosomes.

### d) Effect on Protein and Amino Acid Metabolism

Many balance studies have demonstrated that reduced N retention is often a characteristic feature of gastrointestinal parasitism. This very often results from increased urinary N loss, implying a reduction in the efficiency of utilization of absorbed amino acids. The radio isotopic techniques referred to earlier have shown that high levels of blood protein loss into the gastrointestinal tract are a consistent finding in helminth infections. By using cannulated sheep infected with *T. colubriformis*, demonstrated no differences in the true digestibility of 35S-labelled bacteria in the small intestine or apparently digested N over the whole tract. However, there were plasma protein losses into the small intestine with an increased ileal N outflow and urinary N excretion. Indeed, blood loss accounted for nearly all the additional abomasal N outflow which was seemingly reabsorbed before the terminal ileum. *T. colubriformis* infection, has shown increases in the caecum proximal colon volatile fatty acid and ammonia concentrations and pool sizes and speculated that increased microbial fermentation occurred. Microbial deamination of amino acids would result in an increase in ammonia absorption at the expense of amino acid uptake. Protein digestion is initiated in the abomasum and completed in the proximal small intestine, liberated amino acids being mainly absorbed from the mid-third of the small intestine. *O. ostertagi* infection is thought to bring about pH-mediated limitation on abomasal protein digestion, but in a monospecific infection this is nullified by a compensatory increase in digestion in the small intestine. In addition, the greatly increased plasma loss would have contributed to the increased faecal N loss. Some degradation of the extra N entering the gastrointestinal tract to produce ammonia may have been responsible for increased urinary N loss in infected calves.

Protein also plays important role in the course of trypanosomiasis. The infection caused marked reduction of growth in animals fed a low protein ration whereas the infected and the infected and control animals fed a high protein ration grew at similar rates. It was observed that sheep supplementation with cotton seed cake and maize bran showed a delayed onset of parasitaemia compared to sheep that were only grazing natural grasslands. Fever during infection is associated with increase heat production and increase metabolizable energy for maintenance so that proportion of protein that is used for growth is reduced, as it is metabolized for animals to provide the extra energy required. The increased synthesis of protein occurs at the expense of muscle protein catabolism and loss in body weight.

### e) Effect on Mineral and Vitamin Metabolism

Subclinical parasitism influences bone metabolism through changes in phosphorus and calcium absorption, leading to reduced bone growth. Other changes in micronutrients occur as part of the suite of changes associated with sub-clinical infections, including decreases in copper uptake and changes in sulfate metabolism. There may be release of Cu and resorption and sequestration of Fe and Zn in protein-calorie malnutrition, infection and acute starvation. In addition to vitamin A deficiency Co deficiency may also enhance the susceptibility to disease (also decreases Vit-B12 synthesis). However, the role of micronutrients in for-age selection is relatively undescribed but worthy of investigation.

*Trypanosoma congolense* infection in sheep results in changes in protein metabolism and iron metabolism, and has no, major effects on the concentrations of plasma zinc, copper, calcium, magnesium and inorganic phosphate. Increase serum chloride and calcium concentration in goats infected with *T. vivax* and a gradual fall in the concentration of inorganic phosphate in cattle infected with *T. congolense.* Changes have also been recorded in levels of serum iron, total iron-binding capacity and plasma proteins. A study was designed to follow the changes in the plasma concentrations of zinc, copper, calcium, magnesium, inorganic phosphate, serum iron, and total iron-binding capacity during a course of *T. congolense* infection in sheep.

Appropriate nutrition is the cornerstone of efficient production. By maintaining animal in adequate body condition, you are more likely to achieve your production targets. Good nutrition of animal will maximise immunity and resilience to internal parasites, however this is only one component of a preventive worm control program. If animal fall below critical body condition or graze poor quality or too little pasture, production and financial targets will not be met. Protein is important for lactating and growing young stock. If available pastures are green, protein will usually be adequate; if not, protein supplements will be required to satisfy the protein requirement of stock.

## Conclusion

Although many aspects of the interaction between nutrition and helminth parasites have been established many features remain to be examined. These include the influence of nutrition on established infections, nutritional influences on immune responses to parasites and nutritional interactions with genetic resistance. There is clearly scope for examining the effects of supplementation in greater detail and improvements in supplementation through protected protein technology. The growing interest in host nutrition-parasite interaction per se imply the improving host resilience and/or resistance to infection through management practices by manipulation of nutrients and above all the nutritional health of the host. The implication of changes in host resistance with nutritional state for host productivity need to be better described. Understanding the role of nutrition in improving both resistance and resilience of the host to parasites will be important if producers are to make better use of host acquired immunity and reduce dependence on pesticides for prophylaxis.

The beneficial effect of nutrition, more specifically, the importance of protein nutrition for the maintenance of host immunity to parasitism, the potential use of novel crops and possibilities for biological control have also been discussed. It is now realized that chemical anthelmintic treatment, on its own, may not provide a long-term strategy for managing parasite in ruminants. There is a growing awareness for strategic nutritional supplementation with far reaching consequences, viz. increased production of meat, milk and wool, and also of its quality, growth and reproductive efficiency, parasite control, enhancement of immunity and disease resistance. Good nutritional management of animals will help to control parasites and promote their survival and growth. When used as part of a preventative worm control program, good nutritional management should also help reduce the need for anthelmintic treatment, thereby slowing the development of worm resistance to these chemicals.

## References

Akinbamijo, O.O., Hamminga, B.J., Wensing, Th., Brouwer, B.O., Tolkamp, B.J., Zwart, D. (1992) The effect of Trypanosoma vivax infection in West African dwarf goats on energy and nitrogen metabolism. Veterinary Quaterly. 14. 95-100.

Barger, I.A. (1993) Influence of sex and reproductive status on susceptibility of ruminants to nematode parasites. International Journal of Parasitology. 23. 463-469.

Bedhomme, S., Agnew, P., Sidobre, C., Michalakis, Y. (2004) Virulence reaction norms across a food gradient. Proceedins of Royal Society B. 271(1540).739-744.

Behnke, J.M. et al. (2009) Heligmosomoides bakeri: A model for exploring the biology and genetics of resistance to chronic gastrointestinal nematode infections. Parasitology. 136. 1565-1580.

Bodiga, V.L., Boindala, S., Putcha, U., Subramaniam, K., Manchala R. (2005) Chronic low intake of proteins or vitamins increases the intestinal cpithclila cell apoptosis in Wistar/NIN rats. Nutrition. 21. p. 949-960.

Bown, M.D., Poppi, D.P., Sykes, A.R. (1991) The effect of post-ruminal infusion of protein or energy on the pathophysiology of Trichostrongylus colubriformis infection and body composition in lambs. Australian Journal of Agricultural Research. 42: 253-267.

Bundy, D.A.P., Golden, M.H.N. (1987) The impact of host nutrition on gastrointestinal helminth population. Parasitology. 95. 623-635.

Chandra, R.K. (1993) Nutrition and the immune system. Proceedings of the Nutrition Society. 52.77-84.

Clough, D. et al. (2016) Effects of protein malnutrition on tolerance to helminth infection. Biology letters. 12(6). 20160189.

Coop, R.L., Field, A.C. (1983) Effect of phosphorus intake on growth rate, food intake, and quality of the skeleton of growing lambs infected with the intestinal nematode Trichostrongylus colubriformis. Research in Veterinary Science. 35. 175-81.

Coop, R.L., Huntley, J.F., Smith, W.D. (1995) Effect of dietary protein supplementation on the development of immunity to Ostertagia circumcincta in growing lambs. Research in Veterinary Science. 59. 24-9.

Coop, R.L., Kyriazakis, I. (1999) Nutrition-parasite interaction. Veterinary Parasitology. 84. 187-204.

Cotter, S.C., Simpson, S.J., Raubenheimer, D., Wilson, K. (2011) Macronutrient balance mediates trade-offs between immune function and life history traits. Functional Ecology. 2011. 25(1).186-198.

Cresswell, K.J. et al. (2004) Asia Pacific Journal of Clinical Nutrition. 13(Suppl). S90.

Crompton, D.W., Keymer, A., Singhvi, A., Nesheim, M.C. (1983) Rat dietary fructose and the intestinal distribution and growth of Moniliformis (Acanthocephala). Parasitology. 86. p. 57-71.

De Aguilar-Nascimento, J.E. (2005) The role of macronutrients in gastrointestinal blood flow. In: Curr. Opin. Clinical Nutrition and Metabolic Care. 8. p. 552-556.

De Rosa, A.A., Chirgwin S.R., Fletcher, J., Williams, J.C., Klei, T.R. (2005) Exsheathment of Ostertagia ostertagi infective larvae following exposure to bovine rumen contents derived from low and high roughage diets. Veterinary Parasitology. 20. p. 77-81.

Din, Z. et al. (2018) Parasitic infections, malnutrition and anemia among preschool children living in rural areas of Peshawar, Pakistan. Nutricion Hospitalaria. 35(5). 1145-1152.

Evans, J.W. et al. (2001) Poultry Science. 80. 258.

Fagbemi, B.O. et al. (1990): Veteterinary Parasitology. 35: 29-42.

Faye D., et al. (2005) Acta Tropica. 93. 247-257.

Fekete, S.G., Kellems, R.O. (2007) Interrelationship of feeding with immunity and parasitic infection: A review. Veterinary Medicine. 52. 131-143.

Field, C.J., Johnson, I.R., Schley, P.D. (2002) Nutrients and their role in host resistance to infection. Journal of Leukocyte Biology. 71(1).16-32.

Frost, P.C., Ebert, D., Smith, V.H. (2008) Responses of a bacterial pathogen to phosphorus limitation of its aquatic invertebrate host. Ecology. 89(2). 313-318.

Hailegebriel, T. (2018) Undernutrition, intestinal parasitic infection and associated risk factors among selected primary school children in Bahir Dar, Ethiopia. BMC Infectious Diseases. 18. 394.

Hall, S.R., Knight, C.J., Becker, C.R., Duffy, M.A., Tessier, A.J., Caceres, C.E. (2009) Quality matters: resource quality for hosts and the timing of epidemics. Ecology Letters. 12(2).118-128.

Hall, S.R., Sivars-Becker, L., Becker, C., Duffy, M.A., Tessier, A.J., Caceres, C.E. (2007) Eating yourself sick: transmission of disease as a function of foraging ecology. Ecology Letters. 10(3). 207-218.

Hertzberg, H., Huwyler, U., Kohler, L., Rehbein, S., Wanner, M. (2002) Kinetics of exsheathment of infective ovine and bovine strongylid larvae in vivo and in vitro. Parasitology. 125. p. 65-70.

Holmes, P.H. (1993). Proceedings of Nutrtion Society. 52.113-120.

Hoste, H., Jackson, F., Athanasiadou, S., Thamsborg, S.M., Hoskin, S.O. (2006) The effects of tannin rich plants on parasitic nematodes in ruminants.Trends in Parasitology. 22. p. 253-261.

Houdijk, J.G.M., Kyriazakis, I., Jackson, F., Huntley, J.F., Coop, R.L. (2000) Can an increased metabolizable protein intake affect the periparturient relaxation in immunity against Teladorsagia circumcincta in sheep. Veterinary Parasitology. 91. 43-62.

Kahn, L.P., Knox, M.R., Gray, G.D., Lea, J.M., Walkden-Brown, S.W. (2003) Enhancing immunity to nematode parasites in singlebearing Merino ewes through nutrition and genetic selection.Veterinary Parasitology. 112. 211-225.

Koski, K.G., Scott. M.E. (2001) Gastointestinal nematodes, nutrition and immunity: Breaking the negative spiral. Annual Review of Nutrition. 21. 297-321.

Krist, A.C., Jokela, J., Wiehn, J., Lively, C.M. (2004) Effects of host condition on susceptibility to infection, parasite developmental rate, and parasite transmission in a snail-trematode interaction. Journal of Evolution Biology. 17(1). 33-40.

Kuris, A.M. (1974) Trophic interactions: similarity of parasitic castrators to parasitoids. Quaterly Review of Biology. 49(2).129-148.

Lafferty, K.D. (1999) The evolution of trophic transmission. Parasitology Today. 15(3).111-115.

Lee, K.P., Simpson, S.J., Wilson, K. (2008) Dietary protein-quality influences melanization and immune function in an insect. Functional Ecology. 22(6).1052-1061.

Mac Rae, J.C. (1993). Proceedings of Nutrition Society. 52. 121-131.

Martínez-Ortiz-de-Montellano, C., Vargas-Magaña, J.J., Aguilar-Caballero, A.J. et al. (2007) Combining the effects of supplementary feeding and copper oxide needles improves the control of gastrointestinal nematodes in browsing goats. Veterinary Parasitology. 2007. 146. 66-76.

Mausour, M.M. et al (1992) Veterinary Immunology. 33. 261-269.

Mekonnen, Z. et al. (2014) Schistosoma mansoni infection and undernutrition among school age children in Fincha'a sugar estate, rural part of West Ethiopia. BMC Research Notes. 7. 763.

Nockels, C.F. (1991). Tropical Veterinary Medicine Winter/Spring. 14-17.

Petkevicius, S., Murrell, K.D., Bach Knudsen, K.E., Jorgensen, H., Roepstorff, A., Laue, A., Wachmann, H. (2004) Effects of short chain fatty acids and lactic acids on survival of Oesophagostomum dentatum in pigs. Veterinary Parasitology. 122. p. 293-301.

Petkevicius, S., Thomsen, L.E., Bach Knudsen, K.E., Murrell, K.D., Roepstorff, A. (2007) The effect of inulin on new and pattent infections of Trichuris suis in growing pigs. Parasitology. 134. p. 121-127.

Poppi, D.P. et al. (1986) Nitrogen transactions in the digestive tract of lambs exposed to the intestinal parasite Trichostrongylus colubriformis. British Journal of Nutrition. 55. 593-602.

Poulin, R. (2000). International Journal of Parasitology. 29. 903-914.

Pulkkinen, K., Ebert, D. (2004) Host starvation decreases parasite load and mean host size in experimental populations. Ecology. 85(3). 823-833.

Reynolds, L., Ekwuruke, J.O. (1988) Small Ruminants Research. 1. 175-188.

Reynolds, L.A. et al. (2012) Immunity to the model intestinal helminth parasite Heligmosomoides polygyrus. Seminars in Immunopathology. 34. 829-846.

Robertson, L.J. et al. (1992) Haemoglobin concentrations and concomitant infections of hookworm and Trichuris trichiura in Panamanian primary schoolchildren. Transactions of The Royal Society of Tropical Medicine and Hygiene. 86(6). 654-656.

Roseby, F. B. (1977). Australian Journal of Agricultural Research. 28. 155-164.

Ryder, J.J., Hathway, J., Knell, R.J. (2007) Constraints on parasite fecundity and transmission in an insect-STD system. Oikos. 116(4). 578-584.

Sadd, B.M. (2011) Food-environment mediates the outcome of specific interactions between a bumblebee and its trypanosome parasite. Evolution. 65(10). 2995-3001.

Seppala, O., Liljeroos, K., Karvonen, A., Jokela, J. (2008) Host condition as a constraint for parasite reproduction. Oikos. 117(5).749-753.

Smith, V.H., Jones, T.P., Smith, M.S. (2005) Host nutrition and infectious disease: an ecological view. Advances in Physiology Education. 2005. 3(5). 268-274.

Solomans, N.W., Keusch, G.T. (1981) Nutrition Reviews. 39. 149-161.

Steel, J.W., Syrnons, L.E.A. (1982). Proceedings of the McMuster Animal Health Laboratory 50th Annual Symposium in Parasitology. pp. 235-256.

Sterner, R.W., Elser, J.J. (2002) Ecological stoichiometry: the biology of elements from molecules to the biosphere. Princeton, NJ: Princeton University Press.

Sukhdeo, M.V.K., Bansemir, A.D. (1996) Critical resources that influence habitata selection decisions by gastroinetstinal helminth parasites. International Journal of Parasitology. 26. p. 483-498.

Thompson, S.N., Redak, R.A., Wang, L.W. (2005) Nutrition interacts with parasitism to influence growth and physiology of the insect Manduca sexta L. Journal of Experimental Biology. 208(4). 611-623.

van Houtert, M.F.J. et al. (1995) Dietary protein for young grazing sheep: interactions with gastrointestinal parasitism. Veterinary Parasitology. 60. 283-295.

Verstegen, M.W.A. et al (1991) Journal of Animal Science. 69. 1667.

Yun, C.H. et al. (2000) Intestinal immune responses to coccidiosis. Developmental & Comparative Immunology. 24. 303-324.

# 9

# General Dairy Farm Management to Control Haemoprotozoa Infection

***Deep Narayan Singh and Ranjana Sinha***

*Department of Livestock Farm Complex/Livestock Production Management Bihar Veterinary College, Bihar Animal Sciences University, Patna, Bihar*

Dairy animals are the backbone of animal husbandry. India is the largest milk producer and ranks first in the world with a share of 25% of global milk production. Haemoprotozoan diseases pose significant limitations to the health and production of cattle. It leads to significant losses in the livestock industry worldwide. However, most protozoan parasites in the blood are known to cause anaemia by inducing erythro-phagocytosis. In terms of mortality, reduced milk production and reduced immunity power, hemoprotozoan parasites pose a major threat to the livestock population. Theileria, Babesia, Anaplasma and Trypanosoma are the most important hemoprotozoan diseases of veterinary importance. These diseases affect different livestock species, caused by different species of Trypanosoma, Theileria, Babesia and Anaplasma. Tick-borne hemoprotozoan infections have a significant negative impact on the health and productivity of cattle and result in major losses to the global livestock industry. In tropical and subtropical regions, tick-borne hemoprotozoan infections have a significant impact on animal production. In India, these hemoprotozoan parasites have long posed a serious threat to the survival of exotic and crossbred cattle (Ananda et al., 2009). Haemoprotozoan diseases have deleterious impact on health and production of animals causing death in acute cases, production losses in chronically affected animals which decrease economic share of livestock sector (Bharti et al., 2022)

Ticks are obligate, blood-sucking ectoparasites that prey on cattle (Bishop et al., 2004). Because of their increased ability to survive and grow in hot and humid climates, ticks are a constant source of infection for animals that are susceptible to infection (Chaudhury et al., 2006). It has been estimated that the annual cost of tick control measures and the global losses resulting from diseases carried by ticks could reach several billions (109) US dollars

(McCosker, 1979; Jongejan and Uilenberg, 1994). Without proper control measures, hemoprotozoan diseases have a major negative economic impact due to mortality, decreased milk yield, and decreased animal draft power. This poses a significant barrier to bovine production, which in turn impedes the agricultural and socio-economic development of India (Suryanarayana, 1990; Vahora et al., 2012; Meenakshisundara et al., 2014).

According to the FAO (2004), ticks also reduce fertility and make it more difficult to introduce new cattle breeds. The use of synthetic acaricides to control ticks is common in India (Ghosh et al., 2007). However, relying solely on a single tick control strategy does not guarantee an effective, long-lasting, or sustainable tick management strategy (Nolan, 1990). Indigenous knowledge systems are widely accepted, and in order to create appropriate implementation strategies, it is necessary to identify how health services delivery complements these systems. Therefore, by using and sharing common knowledge (local or indigenous) within the livestock health care system, ectoparasitic infestation can be controlled.

## 1. Haemoprotozoan Disease in Dairy Animals

### Trypanosomosis

Trypanosomosis is a complex disease caused by single-celled flagellate protozoan parasites, trypanosomes, found in the blood and other tissues of vertebrates, including cattle and buffalo. There are variations in the origins, geographic locations, hosts, and clinical features of *Trypanosoma evansi*. It can vary in its hosts, origins, and geographic distribution as well as in its clinical features. It also has a variety of intricate transmission routes, each with a different relative significance based on the host and region. Actually, *T. evansi* can spread vertically, horizontally, iatrogenically, and perorally. Depending on the season, location, and host species, there are various ways that evansi can spread, including by biting insects, sucking insects and vampire bats. In the tropics, trypanosomosis, also referred to as Surra, is one of the main hemo-protozoan diseases that affect both human and animal health (Tiwari et al., 2005; Bossard et al., 2010; Kurup and Tewari, 2012). Surra is most common during the monsoon season when animals are under maximum work stress due to agricultural work. The risk of disease is also increased by additional contributing factors like comorbidities, inadequate nutrition, innate and acquired resistance, parasite pathogenicity, and parasite strain.

Similar to trypanosomes, leeches have the capacity to spread *T. evansi* needs to be looked into, especially for Asia's buffalo leeches (*Hirudinaria manillensis*).

The sources of infection are often animal blood, meat, and milk. Animals that are under stress are more susceptible to the disease.

Sufficient diagnostic tests and distribution data regarding *Trypanosoma evansi* in India are critical for effective surveillance. The degree of knowledge among veterinarians and diagnostic labs regarding *T. evansi* is nearly sufficient; however, rapid identification is hampered by the absence of highly sensitive diagnostic methods. Apart from animal inoculation, microscopic examination is the only diagnostic method with the advantages of high specificity, user-friendliness and lack of cold chain (Singh and Tewari, 2012). However, due to its low sensitivity, it frequently gives a false negative result, which, in the absence of treatment, can even result in the death of animal (Deborggraeve and Buscher, 2010).

Although immune-diagnostic techniques are helpful in the diagnosis of trypanosomosis, their majority have been retrospective surveys that have proven to be ineffective in managing the disease. However, the complement fixation test was used successfully in the control and eradication of Dourine in North America (Watson, 1920) and the diagnosis of surra in buffalo in the Philippines (Randall and Schwartz, 1936). According to Luckins et al (1979), the indirect fluorescent antibody test (IFAT) can detect trypanosome antibodies in both humans and animals with high specificity and sensitivity. But, the cross reactivity between various trypanosoma species and the need for a powerful microscope, however, are two significant issues with IFAT. Other immunodiagnostics followed very often are ELISA (Desquesnes et al., 2013) and card agglutination test (CATT) (Bajyana-Songa et al., 1987). Immunoglobulin IgG is detected by ELISA in cases of established infections, but immunoglobulin IgM can be detected by CATT for early infection detection. It is claimed that a monoclonal anti body-based latex agglutination test, which is straightforward, quick, and affordable in the field, can effectively diagnose surra in domesticated animals (Rayulu et al., 2007; Shyma et al., 2012).

## 2. Theileriosis

Protozoa of the genus Theileria are tick-borne parasites that occur in many mammalian species specially in dairy animals. More than a dozen Theileria species are found and caused disease in cattle, buffalo, sheep and goats. Particularly in domestic animals, some of these have a tendency to circulate with few or no clinical signs, while others can cause severe disease with high rates of morbidity and mortality. *Theileria parva*, the organism that causes East Coast fever/corridor disease, and *T annulata*, the organism that causes tropical theileriosis, are the two that have the highest economic effects on cattle production and reproduction traits. *T. lestoquardi*, *T. uilenbergi* and *T. luwenshuni* are the most virulent species in sheep and goats. Highly virulent species of Theileria not only cause direct losses but also pose a threat to livestock trans-national trade and the introduction of new breeds or improved stock for genetic improvement. The widely distributed *T. orientalis*/ *T. buffeli* group of Theileria is thought to be one of the pathogenic species of Theileria, since 2010, members of this group have been responsible for several cattle outbreaks in Australia, New Zealand, and other nations.

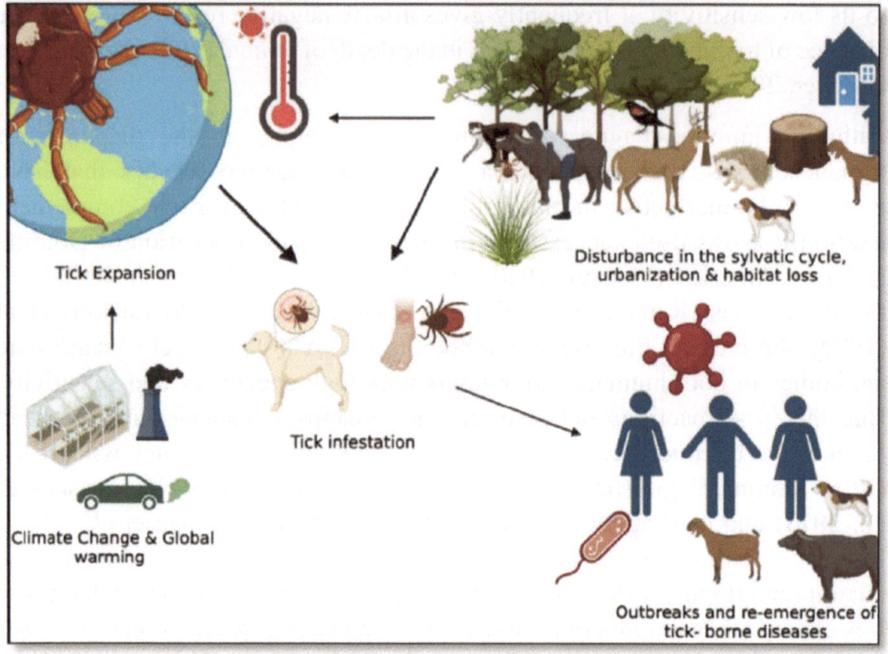


Ticks serve as a biological vector for the spread of theileria, which can spread cross-stadially. It is believed that trans-ovarial transmission does not occurs. Genera of ticks reported to act as vectors include Rhipicephalus (*T. parva*, *T. taurotragi*, *T. ovis*, *T. lestoquardi*), Hyalomma (*T. annulata*, *T. lestoquardi*, *T. separata*), Haemaphysalis (*T. orientalis*, *T. uilenbergi*, *T. luwenshuni*) and Amblyomma (*T. mutans*, *T. velifera*). Theileria species enter the body through tick saliva as sporozoites. Ordinarily, *T. parva* and *T. annulata* only mature after an infected tick attaches to a host, and the tick must be attached for a few days before these organisms are transmitted. Theileria undergoes a complex life cycle, in the mammalian host, involving the replication of schizonts in leukocytes and development of piroplasms in erythrocytes. These Piroplasms stage infect ticks when they feed on the animal's blood. Additionally, theileria can spread mechanically through blood, possibly through biting flies and sucking lice (*Linognathus vituli*). If the temperature is high enough, parva can grow to the infectious stage in ticks present on the ground.

Theileriosis shows anaemia, haemoglobinuria, pyrexia (40.0 °C to 40.1 °C), in-appetence to anorexia and enlarged prescapular lymph nodes as major clinical signs. Heavy infection of *Theileria annulata* in dairy animals also shows pale mucus membranes, salivation and panting as major clinical sign.

### 3. Babesiosis

Among the hemoprotozoan diseases that affect cattle in India, babesiosis is second most important disease that severely affect production and the estimated economic losses is about INR 580.16 crore /year (Vahora et al., 2012). It is acknowledged as a serious problem affecting in bovine species. According to Chakrabarti (2016), in tropical and sub-tropical regions of the world, including India, the economic losses occur in the form of animal deaths, reduced productivity, and decreased working efficiency.

Bovine babesiosis, a tick-borne disease that affects cattle and buffalo in tropical and subtropical regions of Africa, Australia, America, Asia and India, it is caused by the intraerythrocytic hemoprotozoa Babesia bigemina transmitted by a variety of tick species.

*Babesia bovis* has been reported from Europe, Africa, Asia, and the East; Babesia argentina is found in southeast Asia and Australia, as well as from Mexico down through Latin America. *Babesia bigemina* distributed in cattle throughout Central and South America, Europe, Africa, Australia, and Asia. Walker and Edward in 1927 was reported first time Babesiosis in India. *Babesia bigemina* and *Babesia bovis* species typically found in tropical and subtropical regions (Radostits et al., 2010). In India, *Babesia bigemina* is the main species commonly found in bovines (Ruprah, 1985). The ticks *Riphicephalus microplus* and *Riphicephalus annulatus* are the natural carriers of the disease, transferring it from sick to healthy animals (Murrell et al., 2001). Both domestic and wild animals are susceptible to babesiosis, and have ability to evade the immune systems, characterized by extensive erythrocytic lysis, which results in anorexia, pyrexia, anaemia, icterus, haemoglobinuria, decreased milk supply and even death. The main cause of pathogenicity of high percent of mortality in non-immune cattle-herd infected with haemoprotozoan diseases is marked anaemia.

Anaemia is the primary reason of the high percentage of death in non-immune cow herds affected with hemoprotozoan illnesses. The primary method of preventing babesiosis in enzootic area is to eliminate the tick vector by regularly dipping cattle in an acaricidal solution at intervals of two weeks or less, depending on the local ecology of vector species.

## 4. Anaplasmosis

The most important species in cattle is *Anaplasma marginale*, which is found throughout tropical, sub-tropical and even temperate regions. Early in the century, *A. centrale*, a less virulent species, was also found in South Africa. Despite the immunological differences, they share several common antigens thus A. centrale is widely used to immunize against *A. marginale*. The morphological difference between the two species is in the site within the red cell. A. marginale is often spread *via* ticks, of which multiple species have been identified. Other than ticks, biting insects can be important in mechanical transmission under certain conditions, especially large tabanid flies during seasonal outbreaks. Most transmission trials with smaller insects, including mosquitoes and stable flies, have had negative findings. While reports of transmission through the egg have occasionally been made, most workers have had negative results, and the majority of transmission appears to be transstadial. Although field data implicates *Boophilus* spp. as important vectors, but carefully controlled transmission trials have yielded negative results. The basic Babesia-Boophilus model can be used to understand the epizootiology of anaplasmosis, in which Boophilus species serve as the main vectors. It was expected that since they are single-host ticks, the transmission method would be transovarial, via the egg. However, for transstadial transmission experiments in Madagascar and Australia have yielded positive results with *B. microplus*; a small percentage of ticks appear to transfer spontaneously from one host animal to another during the tick's life cycle (Uilenberg, 1970; Connell and Hall, 1972; Leatch, 1973). It has still to be determined whether transfer of one-host ticks from one host individual to another occurs frequently enough in the field to explain the vector role of *Boophilus*. (controversial statement)

Young calves are less susceptible to infection than adults, where chances of anaemia do occur occasionally when they are in enzootic conditions, i.e., there is not much of a disease problem but become important in epizootic situations.

Although it has been demonstrated that some antibodies are transferred from the immune dam to the calf through the colostrum, it is still unclear whether protective antibodies are also present against anaplasmosis. It also has to be shown unambiguously that indigenous zebu breeds are more resistant to anaplasmosis than crossbred and exotic cattle breeds. Once an animal recovers from an infection, the infection most likely stays with it for the rest of its life, making the animal immune to the adverse consequences of further infections. It is possible that immunologically diverse strains may exist in field condition and may having different degrees of virulence but their significance in the field is uncertain.

## Management strategies to Prevent Haemoprotozoan Disease

1. **Hygiene in animal house:** Housing is an important activity of all modern animal welfare programmes. Scientific animal housing is necessary to secure the most benefits from livestock in terms of productivity and services to the humanity. A clean shelter improves the animal's comfort level in addition to having positive benefits on its health. Maintaining good hygiene helps protect animals from bacterial, viral, and parasite infections as well as associated diseases. Animals need to be kept in hygienic circumstances, especially, the type of weather and severe climate conditions that they live in. Good sanitation procedures are essential in animal housing to prevent the spread of haemoprotozoan disease to other animals.
2. **Sanitation of animal houses:** According to the World Health Organization, environmental sanitation is the management of all components in the physical environment of humans and animals that negatively impact their growth, well-being, and ability to survive. The physical environment includes the non-living things and physical factors affecting the animals, such as air, ventilation, lighting, noise, climate and water. The term "sanitation" refers to the entire farm that managing an animal's surroundings in order to prevent disease and improve health. One of the main issues with maintaining sanitation in animal houses is the importance of environmental sanitation for both protecting and promoting the animal and worker's health and safety. Eliminating additional environmental variables that are detrimental to the health of humans and animals.

Moist manure or other wet decomposing organic materials are where flies and ticks near dairy buildings. In unhygienic conditions, it is unrealistic to expect an insecticide to keep flies under control. A comprehensive program for sanitation is necessary to control fly populations in and around livestock facilities.

(a) Remove all manure from livestock pens as frequently as possible. Special attention are needed for bull shed, calf shed, milch shed, dry shed, and heifer shed that include animals. Cleaning these pens once in a day. Fly development is decreased when sawdust is used as animal bedding rather than other materials in calf pen. More hygienic cattle barns have fewer fly issues.

(b) Either stack this trash and cover with a black plastic tarp, or spread the manure thinly outside so that fly eggs and larvae will be killed by drying.

(c) Remove any organic matter accumulations that can attract flies from the farm, such as old wet hay or straw bales, damp litter, silage seepage spots, and manure stacks. Wet feed remaining at the ends of mangers will breed flies.

(d) Ensure that barnyards have sufficient drainage. Ensure that barnyards have sufficient drainage. Lower areas in livestock yards can be eliminated by using clean gravel and other fill. Proper grading and covering with brick can reduced wet barnyards. Keep water troughs and hydrants leak-free.

### 3. Ventilation

Animal houses must have good ventilation in order to replace stale air with fresh air. Inadequate ventilation in animal housing results in warmer, more humid stagnant air that condenses on surfaces, floors, and bedding, making it uncomfortable for the animals.

It is generally caused by uneven distribution of animals makes animals more concentrated at certain areas and accumulates excreta and expired air in certain pockets. All those factors, such as dust, particulate matter, ammonia, other gasses and pathogenic germs carried by animals, aggravates respiratory and gastrointestinal diseases, mastitis, and other infections. High humidity with high temperature during the rainy season is favourable for the spread of various infections.

### 4. Cleaning of Animals and Their Environment

Physical cleaning removes biological material and excreta from the animal's body and surroundings. The surface should be evidently cleaned by using warm, soapy and clean water. Frequent cleaning can reduce offensive odours in shelters and adjacent areas. It helps in avoiding a number of diseases that affect farms and animals. Using a possible disinfectant after cleaning can help to eliminate hazardous biological entities from the environment and aid in the elimination of harmful pathogen. Applying a germicidal chemical on the surface is necessary for effective sanitation. Products of both detergent and disinfection must be used for effective removal of germs. Almost all disinfectants used in shelters are rendered ineffective if not sprayed to a clean surface because organic material like excreta, saliva, urine, sneeze marks, regular dirt and left over feed can inactivate them to some degree.

## 5. Managemental Strategies to Control of Ticks

One of the main challenges for dairy and others domestic animals in tropical environments is tick infestation. Ticks transmit many parasitic diseases in dairy and other domestic animals as well as human beings. It adversely affects physiology of animal leads to reduction in production and reproduction trait of dairy and meat animals. Its infestation also causes skin diseases. Traditionally, farmers used chemical control, but this method is unidirectional. By spraying insecticide on animals' bodies, they are able to kill ticks and other ectoparasites but not control them in surrounding environment. Ticks may hide in cracks, fissures in and around animal sheds beneath stones, boulders, damp regions and waste material locations.

i) **Rearing under tick proof shed:** Dairy animal's shelters should be as tick-proof as feasible, especially when keeping exotic and crossbred animals, which are more prone to tick infestation than native cattle and buffaloes. There should not have any cracks and crevices in the shed because that is where ticks hide and breed. Caulking of the walls of the animal's sheds is an inexpensive measure that significantly reduces the tick burden. An acaricide should be encircle the entire building. Heaps of dung cakes and stacks of bricks is the breeding places for the ticks in animal sheds and they should be remove and repaired regularly.

iii) **Burning of the wastes near the walls under animal sheds:** Although female ticks usually lay their eggs in the cracks and fissures in the walls of animal sheds, the load of ticks on animals can be efficiently reduced by scraping farm waste (faeces, feed waste, etc.) against the walls of empty paddocks and slowly burning it over a period of one or two days. It is advice to repeat these practices on a regular basis. Use of this procedure should only occur after all appropriate safety measures have been taken.

iii) **Separate housing of cattle and buffaloes:** Cattle, especially those with exotic blood such as crossbred and exotic cattle are more susceptible to tick infection than buffaloes. Buffaloes don't usually carry cattle ticks unless they are in stress. They are not the usual host of cattle ticks. When cattle and buffaloes are mixed together, the buffaloes sometimes also suffer from heavy tick infestation. Cattle and buffaloes should therefore have separate housing.

iv) **Quarantine:** Quarantine is the segregation of healthy animals especially animals being brought into the herd for the first time, which have been exposed to the risk of infection from those animals, which are healthy and unexposed to the risk of infection. It is not advisable to immediately add recently purchased animals with the farm's current livestock. Animals should undergo a comprehensive screening for parasite infestation throughout the quarantine period using faecal examination, and deworming should be done properly. Before adding new animals to the herd, if there are ticks on their body, they should be treated with acaricides to rid them of the ticks. On the 25th or 26th day, the animals should also be sprayed or dipped to get rid of any ectoparasites that may have been present.

v) **Pasture management:** Pasture management is a sustainable method of controlling tick populations, its application is not common in India due to the small land holdings of many livestock farmers.

However, this approach remains a feasible choice that can be implemented in cooperative farming where animals have access to grazing space or in organized livestock farms (India has 257 government-controlled livestock farms and numerous dairy cooperatives). All that is required for this approach are great fencing and managemental skills. The most significant range legume for the humid to semi-arid tropics in India is Stylosanthes. A diversified group of species, the Stylosanthes genus is widely distributed in tropical, subtropical, and temperate regions. For the production of animals, it is widely used in pastoral, agro-pastoral, and silvi-pastoral systems (Chandra et al., 2006). In addition to their ability to attract ticks, these features will enhance the nutrition of animals. Government policies supporting the cultivation of certain kind of grasses by offering lower seed cost and inspiring farmers through extension education could help reduce the spread of diseases carried by ticks. A livestock farmer can produce high-quality milk and meat at a lower price without using a lot of pesticides by simply managing the pasture, which includes rotating grazing, planting tick-trapping gasses, and spelling the pasture. These low-cost methods contribute to a tick-free or tick-lower-than-before environment by reduced use of acaricides.

vi) **Rotational grazing in pasture:** The pasture spelling and rotational grazing has dramatically reduced the population of one-host ixodid ticks or *Boophilus microplus*, on Australian dairy farms (David, 2005). Tick population can be reduced with significantly fewer acaricidal treatments if cattle are placed on spelled (i.e., divided) pastures early in winter when the ticks are producing few or no progeny and then alternatively used at every 4-monthly intervals. Duration of the spelling period varies from two to three months in summer and three to four months in winter, but these intervals need to be determined for each area. Pasture spelling is not very useful in developing countries like India because most pastures and ranges are owned communally. Pasture spelling and rotation are not very successful methods of controlling multi-host ixodid ticks (e.g., *Hyalomma anatolicum anatolicum*) or *Argasid* ticks because nymphs and adults can survive for long periods of time without feeding.

vii) **Manual removal of ticks:** In areas where there are relatively few tick-infested cattle or buffaloes, farmers typically physically remove the ticks during milking. After being removed, ticks are destroyed by placing them next to a combustible dung cake. Ticks can be manually removed by grasping them near the animal's body with the forefingers, then twisting them counterclockwise. Tick eradication by hand is enjoyable for cattle.

When physically removing the tick, one should consider the possible risk that these ticks are possible hazardous to humans. The most significant and lethal known human pathogen is the Crimean-Congo Hemorrhagic Fever (CCHF) virus, which is typically connected to ticks belonging to the Hyalomma genus. Within the geographical range of Rhipicephalus appendiculatus, CCHF is extensively distributed. Thus, both conventional farmers and researchers collecting ticks for study should be informed about the possibility of CCHF virus transmission associated with manual tick removal. Ticks should never be squashed between the fingers, instead of they should be extracted using forceps (OIE, 2004).

Viii) **Biological control strategies for ticks:** Ticks have numerous natural enemies, but only a few species have been assessed as tick biocontrol agents. The most promising entomopathogenic fungus appear in several commercial strains of *Metarhizium anisopliae* and *Beauveria bassiana* are now available for the control of some crop pests. The practical significance of parasitoid wasps and entomopathogenic nematodes in the limited pragmatic role in tick control. Predators such as ants, spiders, shrews, birds and rodents, accomplish a portion of tick management. Ox-peckers Buphagus species feed on ticks from the bodies of infected animals, and because certain birds prey on ticks, cattle and buffaloes tied under trees throughout the summer months typically have low tick burdens. Raising poultry chicks in cattle barns greatly reduces the number of ticks on the infested animals because the young birds, in particular, take up ticks from the bodies of the cattle as well as from ticks moving around the barn. Mixed poultry and dairy husbandry poses a risk of infectious diseases such as salmonellosis and crytococcosis, as well as significant feed waste for cattle.

## 6. Breeding of Dairy Animal for Tick Resistance

The best way to reduce tick management costs is to choose animals that are more resistant to ticks. A genetic improvement program targeting tick resistance breed and gene must be used for selection purpose that can pass resistance gene to their progeny, lowering a population's susceptibility in a particular enzootic area. As a result, the parasite load in the area would decrease, which would lessen the need for chemical control measures.

The existence of genetic resistance to ticks in a particular group is the true obstacle in the selection process for enhanced host resistance. Finding the animal breed that is naturally resistant is one of the easiest methods to accomplish this. However, numerous objectives of any breeding effort can be attained with minimal additional investment if the tick resistance trait is linked to production and reproduction trait.

Studies conducted by Frisch (1981) and Burrow et al. (1991) have demonstrated that populations susceptible to tick and worm infestations develop resistance through selection favouring fast growth when these parasites are present. Several studies have shown that there is a low to non -significant genetic correlation between tick count and a variety of productive, adaptive, and pubertal traits (Davis, 1993; David, 2005; Prayaga et al., 2009). According to Prayaga and Henshall (2005), tick resistance is unlikely to be genetically improved by selection for growth in tropical conditions. Some workers have said that there is variation in host resistance to ticks and this may be genetically transmitted to their offspring. They have also estimated the heritability for resistance to ticks. Cattle breeds selected for their tick resistance character had shown significant improvements to develop cattle breeds that are both productive and resistant to ticks. Heritability of tick resistance varies from very low to high (Alencar et al., 2005). This variation in heritability is depends upon method of genetic evaluation, trait considered, permanent environment effect and additive genetic variation for resistance, which is intrinsic to each studied population. The differences in heritability may be due to variation in tick resistance expression across various studies. According to Utech et al. (1978), resistance in Brahman cattle seems to be a dominant trait when considering interbreeds. In an Australian Illawarra Shorthorn herd, resistance has increased from 89.2 to 99% over years of selection. In this herd, the progeny's resistance improved concurrently from 93.7 to 97.7%, indicating that the breeding and selection of cows and bulls led to a genetic improvement in the progeny's resistance (Utech and Wharton 1982). Australian Friesian Sahiwal, which have been developed with acceptable levels of milk production and bulls with high tick resistance in a tropical environment. Mackinnon (1990) has shown that selection in tropical beef breeds may readily affect tick resistance. Despite the successes achieved in Australia, in selection against tick resistance, where they are concerned with only one tick species, there is less anticipation from other regions of the world, especially in Asia and Africa. DeCastro and Newson (1993) suggested that selection for cattle lines or breeds that possess enhanced genetic resistance against ticks is a desirable prospect. After initial exposure, the native breeds of Asia and Africa, Zebu (*Bos indicus*; e.g., Sahiwal) and Sanga (*Bos taurus* × *Bos indicus*) cattle, typically develop strong resistance against ixodid ticks. In order to control tick populations, breeders are using Zebu breeds and their crosses to produce tick resistance in the following generation. Since the introduction of Zebu livestock, especially Sahiwal cattle, the control of Boophilus microplus on the Australian continent has undergone an enormous change. According to a study on genetically modified animals and vaccinations against ticks, Brossard (1998) revealed that some members of the herd are more resistant to ticks than others, regardless of breed.

According to Bonsma (1983) the following elements underlie Zebu cattle's tick resistance and repellency. High skin vascularity and well-developed panniculus muscle, a sensitive pilomotor nervous system that moves their hides at the slightest provocation, thick movable hides covered in short, straight, non-medulated hair (the skin of European breeds is thin and covered in woolly hair), a high density of sweat glands, and an effective erector pili muscle that causes the hair to stand up in response to provocation from flies, ticks, and other insects while also stimulating the production of sebum, a tick repellent.

## 7. Fly Control

Flies are a major cause of disease and economic loss of dairy farmer all around the world. All together, they are known to have contributed to the spread of many diseases, such as cholera, typhoid fever, diarrhoea, leprosy, tuberculosis and others diseases. They are also responsible for significant reductions in the production as well as quality of livestock and poultry product. Now a day, fly control is a major concern in farms because these modern farm practices often provide an ideal breeding habitat for flies.

The disposal of manure and urine on a regular basis at a sufficient distance from the cattle shed may help in fly control in the farm. Drainage from farm should not be stagnant and covered during its way. Smoking the shed with raw leaves, preferably neem leaves, especially in the evening would help in reduce fly in the farm. Fly repellents can be used in appropriate concentration.

## 8. Vaccination of Animal

There are presently four vaccinations against hemoprotozoan diseases: theileriosis, babesiosis, anaplasmosis, and babesiosis use in Israel. These vaccines contain live, attenuated parasites that are obtained from the blood of infected, splenectomized calves (*Babesia bigemina, B. bovis*, and *Anaplasma centrale*) or from cell culture (*Theileria annulata* and *Besnoitia besnoiti*). The vaccine production begins with the use of cryopreserved master seed. Quality control performed during the preproduction period is particularly important with blood-derived vaccines. Sterility, potency (viability of immunizing organisms), safety (degree of attenuation), and efficacy (ability to defend against virulent parasite stock) are the four components of post-production quality control. All vaccines are stored and dispatched to the field in a concentrated frozen state. The culture-derived vaccines are safe for all type of cattle, irrespective of age or physiological condition, whereas the blood-derived vaccines are recommended mostly for young animals, the age limit varying with the type of vaccine and breed of cattle. The infectivity of blood-derived immunizations is tested by titration in susceptible cattle. The anti-theilerial vaccine's viability is evaluated by in vitro plating efficiency following thawing.

The *T. annulata* attenuated cultured schizont vaccine is safe for use in cows of all breeds. In areas where tick exposure is continuous, immunity can be boosted in areas where tick exposure is highest, revaccination every three years is recommended.

Tick-derived sporozoites and a long-acting tetracycline formulation are injected together to provide protection against *T. parva*. This procedure provides long-lasting immunity for life.

There are vaccinations for anaplasmosis that are both live and killed vaccine are available, but none of them totally prevent against infection. More research is being done to develop vaccines that work better for different population living in different environment.

## References

Alencar M.M., Fraga, A.B. and Silva, A.M. (2005). Adaptac¸a ˜o de genotipos a ambientes tropicais: resistencia a` mosca-doschifres (Haemato bia irritans, Linnaeus) eao carrapato (Boophilus microplus, Canestrini) em diferentes geno´tipos bovinos. [Genotype adaptation to tropical environments: cattle resistance to horn fly (Haematobia irritans, Linnaeus) and to cattle tick (Boophilus microplus, Canestrini) in different cattle genotypes]. Agrociencia 9:579–585

Ananda, K.J., D'Souza, P.E. and Puttalakshmamma, G.C. (2009). Prevalence of haemo-protozoan diseases in cross bred cattle in Bangalore North. Vet. World, 2: 15-16.

Bajyana-Songa, E., Hamers-Casterman, C., Hamers, R., Pholpark, M., Pholpark, S., Leidl, K, Tangchaitrong, S., Chaichanopoonpol, I., Vitoorakool, C. and Thirapataskum, T. (1987). The use of a card agglutination test (Testryp CATT) for use in detection of T. evansi infection: A comparison with other trypanosomiasis diagnostic tests under field conditions in Thailand. Ann. Soc. Belg. Med. Trop., 67: 137-148.

Bharti, V., Pilania, P.K., Choudhary, P. and Joshi, S.P. (2022). Prevalence Rate of Haemoprotozoan Infection and Assessment of Associated Risk Factors in Dairy Animals from Bikaner Region of Rajasthan, India. J. Anim. Res., 12(01): 69-74.

Bishop, R., Musoke, A., Morzaria, S., Gardner, M., Nene, V. (2004). "Theileria: parasites Intracellular protozoan of wild and domestic ruminants transmitted by Ixodid ticks". Parasitology, 129(7): S271 S283

Bonsma, J. (1983). Livestock Production: A global approach. CBS Publishers and Distributors, Delhi, India, pp: 45-46.

Bossard, G., Boulange, A., Holzmuller, P., Thévenon, S., Patrel, D. and Authie, E. (2010) Serodiagnosis of bovine trypanosomosis based on HSP70/BiP inhibition ELISA. Vet. Parasitol., 173(1-2): 39-47.

Brossard, M. (1998). The use of vaccines and genetically resistant animals in tick control. In: Genetic Resistance to Animal Diseases. Blancou, J. (ed.), Scientific and Technical Review, Office International des Epizooties (OIE), Paris, France, 17(1): 188-199.

Burrow. H.M., Gulbransen, B., Johnson, S.K., Davis, G.P., Shorthose, W.R. and Elliott, R.F. (1991). Consequences of selection for growth and heat resistance on growth, feed conversion efficiency, commercial carcass traits and meat quality of zebu crossbred cattle. Aust J Agric Res 42:1373–1383.

Chakrabarti, A. (2016). A Textbook of Preventive Veterinary Medicine. 2nd edn. Kalyani Publishers, New Delhi.

Chandra, A., Pathak, P.S. and Bhatt, R.K. (2006). Stylosanthes research in India: prospects and challenges ahead. Curr Sci, 90: 915-921.

Chaudhury, S., Hossain, M.A., Barua, S.R. and Islam, S. (2006). Occurrence of common blood parasites of cattle in Serajgong Sadar area of Bangladesh. Bangladesh. J. Vet. Med. 4(2):143–145.

Connell, M. and Hall, W.T.K. (1972). Transmission of Anaplasma marginale by the cattle tick Boophilus microplus. Aust. vet. J., 48: 477.

David, S. (2005). Ticks. In: The Merck Veterinary Manual. 9th Ed., Kahn, C. M. (ed.). Merck and Co., Inc., Whitehouse Station, New Jersey USA, pp: 749-764.

Davis, G.P. (1993). Genetic-parameters for tropical beef-cattle in northern Australia: a review. Aust J Agric Res 44:179–198.

Deborggraeve, S. and Buscher, P. (2010). Molecular diagnostics for sleeping sickness: What is the benefit for the patient? Lancet Infect. Dis., 10: 433-439.

DeCastro, J. J. and Newson, R. M. (1993). Host resistance in cattle tick control. Parasitol. Today, 9: 13-17.

Desquesnes, M., Dargantes, A., Lai, D.H., Lun, Z.R., Holzmuller, P. and Sathaporn, J. (2013) Trypanosoma evansi and surra: A review and perspectives on transmission, epidemiology and control, impact, and zoonotic aspects. Biomed. Res. Int., 2013: 321237.

FAO (2004). Mechanisms of acaricide resistance management and integrated parasite control in ruminants- guidelines, Module I-Ticks, Acaricide Resistance, Diagnosis, Management and Prevention, Rome,Italy.

Food and Agricultural Organisation of the United Nation (FAO) (1984). Ticks and tick-borne disease control. A practical field manual, Vol.1. Tick Control.FAO, Rome. 299pp.

Frisch, J.E. (1981). Factors affecting the resistance to ecto- and endoparasites of cattle in tropical areas and the implications for selection. In: IAEA (ed) Isotopes and radiation in parasitol ogy IV. Panel Proceeding Series. Pub. 572, Vienna, pp 17–32.

Ghosh, S., Azhahianambi P, Yadav MP (2007) Upcoming and future strategies of tick control: a review. J. Vector. Borne. Dis. 44: 79–89.

Jongejan, F. and Uilenberg, G. (1994). Ticks and control methods. Rev. sci. tech. off. int. Epiz., 13(4);1201-1226.

Kurup, S.P. and Tewari, A.K. (2012) Induction of protective immune response in mice by a DNA vaccine encod ing Trypanosoma evansi beta tubulin gene. Vet. Parasitol., 187: 9-16.

Leatch, G. 1973. Preliminary studies on the transmission of Anaplasma marginale by Boophilus microplus. Aust. vet. J., 49: 16–19.

Luckins, A.G., Boid, R., Rae, P., Mahmoud, M.M., EI-Malik, K.H. and Gray, A.R. (1979). Sero diagnosis of infection with Trypanosoma evansi in camels in the Sudan. Trop. Anim. Health Prod., 11: 1-12.

Mackinnon, M.J. (1990). Genetic relationships between growth and fertility in tropical beef cattle. In: Blair HT (ed) Proceedings of 8th conference of the Australian Association of Animal Breeding and Genetics. Hamilton and Palmerston North, New Zealand.

McCosker, P.J. (1979). Global aspects of the management and control of ticks of veterinary importance, In Recent advance in acarology (J. Rodriguez, ed.). Academic press, New York, vol. 2, 45-53.

Meenakshisundaram, A., Anna, T. and Malmarugan, S. (2014). Concomitant Theileria annulata and Anaplasma marginale infections in a cross bred dairy herd. Ind. J. Vet & Anim. Sci. Res., 43(6); 422-425.

Murrell, A., Campbell, N.J.H. and Barker, S.C. (2001). A total evidence phylogeny of ticks provides insights into evolution of life cycles and biogeography. Mol. Phylogenet. Evol.: 21: 244-258.

Nolan, J. (1990). Acaricide resistance in single & multi-host ticks and strategies for control. Parasitology 32:145–153.

OIE (2004). Manual of diagnostic tests and vaccines for terrestrial animals.5th Ed.,Office Internationale des Epizooties, Paris, France.

Prayaga, K.C., Corbet, N.J., Johnston, D.J., Wolcott, M.L., Fordyce, G. and Burrow, H.M. (2009). Genetics of adaptive traits in heifers and their relationship to growth, pubertal and carcass traits in two tropical beef cattle genotypes. Anim Prod Sci 49:413–425.

Prayaga, K.C. and Henshall, J.M. (2005). Adaptability in tropical beef cattle: genetic parameters of growth, adaptive and temperament traits in a crossbred population. Aust J Exp Agric 45:971–983.

Radostits, O.M., Gay, C.C., Hinchcliff, K.W., and Constable, P.D. (2010). Veterinary Medicine. A textbook of the diseases of cattle, horses, sheep, pigs and goats, 10th edn. Pp. 2045 2050.

Randall, R. and Schwartz, S.C. (1936). A survey for the incidence of surra in the Philippine islands. Vet. Bull. US Army, 30: 99-108.

Rayulu, V.C., Singh, A. and Chaudhri, S.S. (2007). Monoclonal antibody based immunoassays for detection of circulating antigens of Trypanosoma evansi in buffaloes. Ital. J. Anim. Sci., 6: 907-910.

Ruprah, N. S. (1985). Text Book of Clinical Protozoology, Oxanian Press Pvt. Ltd. New Delhi, Pp 287-304.

Shyma, K.P., Gupta, S.K., Singh, A. and Chaudhri, S.S. (2011) Latex agglutination test for detection of trypanosomosis in equines. J. Vet. Parasitol., 25(2): 132-134.

Singh, V. and Tewari, A.K. (2012) Bovine surra in India: An update. Rumin. Sci., 1(1): 1-7.

Suryanarayana, C. (1990). A review of haematological and biochemical picture in haemoprotozoan disease of cattle. Liv. Adv., 15:15.

Tewari, A.K., Rao, J.R., Mishra, A.K. and Yadav, M.P. (2005) Recent trends in the diagnosis of trypanosomosis (surra) in domesticated animals. Proc. Natl. Acad. Sci. India, 75(B): 121-133.

Uilenberg, G. (1970). Note sur les babésioses et l'anaplasmose des bovins à Madagascar. IV. Note additionellesurla transmission. Rev. Élev. Méd. vét. Pays trop., 23: 309–312.

Utech, K.B.W., Seifert, G.W. and Wharton, R.H. (1978). Breeding Australian Illawarra Shorthorn cattle for resistance to Boophilus microplus. 1. Factors affecting resistance. Aust J Agric Res 29:411–422.

Utech, K.B.W. and Wharton, R.H. (1982). Breeding for resistance to Boophilus microplus in Australian Illawarra Shorthorn and Brahman 9 Australian Illawarra Shorthorn cattle. Aust Vet J 58: 41–46.

Vahora, S.P., Patel, J.V., Parel, B.B., Patel, S.B., Umale, R.H. (2012). Seasonal incidence of haemoprotozoan disease in crossbred cattle and buffalo in Kaira and Anand district of Gujarat, India. Vet World, 5(4): 223–225.

Walker, G.K. and Edward, J.T. (1927) Some Diseases of Cattle in India. Government of India, Calcutta. p29.

Watson, E.A. (1920). Dourine in Canada. History, Research, Suppression. Dominion of Canada, Department of Agriculture.

# Index